Just Because
I Am Old

A Practical and Theological Guide to Caring

JAMES A. STINSON

Produced by:

FriesenPress

Suite 300 – 852 Fort Street
Victoria, BC, Canada V8W 1H8

www.friesenpress.com

Distributed to the trade by The Ingram Book Company

Table of Contents

To Barbara

*Who is growing old with me and helps me
remember 'the best is yet to be.'*

Just Because I Am Old

A Practical and Theological Guide To Caring

Preface

A strange thing happened to me on the way to becoming a senior citizen! My views began to change! Always one to enjoy the older members of the churches I served as the pastor, I nonetheless developed a view that was both wrong and destructive of them. For years I treated them with "kid gloves," unconsciously assuming because they were "old" they were fragile and should not have to deal with the give and take of everyday life. I excused some behavior, which I would never have tolerated from a younger person, on the grounds that "they are old." In retrospect, it was demeaning to them since it did not allow for them to be seen as complete human beings, able and needing to interact with others in mutually acceptable ways.

While I do not think I ever talked down to them, I know I did not always credit them with the same wisdom my "young and vibrant" members possessed. More than once I would subtly dismiss a critique of a new proposal by an older person because "old people just have difficulty accepting new ideas." I wonder how many dumb ideas I've pursued because of this bias. Older people do not always reject new ideas! Young people do not always have the best ideas! It was my assumption about age being a time of frailty and less ability that at times kept me from seeing this in my younger years.

Now I don't feel guilty about this particularly. It is safe to say that many, if not most, people share these assumptions at some point in their lives. Our culture, with its adoration of youth, with its denial of the aging process, with its ever burgeoning "be young again" advertising mentality, and a host of other misguided thoughts, has conditioned us to think in these terms. We have been led to see aging as a disease to be denied for as long as possible! We have been taught to be caring for the aging, but not always to see them as whole people. We have learned so many things about aging that need to be examined and unlearned.

Fortunately I had a good teacher who forced me, even before I recognized I was doing so, to look again at my assumptions about aging. She did so by her very presence and by the way she lived her life. And more fortunately she lived with me, subtly influencing the way I engaged in ministry with the older adults in my congregations. When my father died and it became financially impossible for my mother to live alone, my wife and I extended the invitation to her to join our household. Little did we know that she would survive for another twenty six years, living nearly three years longer than my wife. Time after time she would demonstrate a wisdom that I only now fully appreciate. Two simple examples are as clear today as they were when they occurred.

One was the night my wife died, my mother, who was already showing early signs of dementia, came down the stairs and said she wanted to talk to me. "Not now Mom," I thought to myself, "just give me a day or two to deal with whatever it is you want to say." But that is not what I said. Instead I simply listened. "Jim, you've done all you could for Judie. You were a good husband. Tomorrow, you move on and let God take care of her and you." Words of love! Words of wisdom! Words I desperately needed to hear! How often I have wondered if I would ever have heard them had I followed my instinct and assumed an old woman, already in dementia, had nothing of value to say! How grateful I am that my bias did not get in the way of listening to a voice that offered a simple, yet eloquent wisdom.

James Andrew Stinson

The other was the day she said my brother, who lived on the other side of the country and did not get to see her very often, had arranged for her to go to the Holy Land and to Italy. She was already well into her seventies, had trouble walking at times, had increasing transient ischemic attacks, and at times was forgetful. I was annoyed at my brother for thinking she could make this trip. I was annoyed at her for thinking she would accept the offer. I was annoyed at myself for feeling the need to tell her she should not go. Quietly, but firmly, she said: "I'm going! I know you're worried about me but there's really nothing to worry about. The worst that can happen is I'll get sick. There are doctors over there as well as here. And if I die, I'll die having a good time. I don't intend to stop living just because I'm old." Again words of wisdom from an older adult that influenced me then and influences me now.

We are too quick to dismiss the aging, making assumptions that may not be correct, assumptions that may convince the very ones we love to "stop living just because they are old." This insight shared in so many ways by a mother who lived a full, active life, being president of the Senior Citizen's Club, a leader at the Senior Center, an active participant and contributor in the life of the Church has stayed with me through the years. As has the lives of countless senior church members, equally vibrant, the value of which was enhanced by her subtle example!

So it was not all that surprising to me when, in 2002, I took early retirement as an ordained minister in the United Methodist Church for the purpose of becoming the full time Director of Spiritual Life for The United Methodist Homes, based in Shelton, CT. The United Methodist Homes owns and operates three communities in Connecticut. One is a continuing care retirement village in Shelton, and two are assisted living facilities in Newington and Farmington respectively. In these places I have learned, and am still learning, how to implement the insight: "You don't stop living just because you are old." I have wrestled and am wrestling with the practical applications of that in doing ministry with and for older adults. As I began pursuing this new vocation, I was asked to become the consultant on Older Adult Ministries for the New York Annual Conference of the United Methodist Church. Part of that responsibility includes writing regularly for our Conference newspaper, *The Vision.* The responses to these articles have helped me understand that this wrestling is taking place in many hearts across the Conference and across the country. Letters and phone calls from people I know, and from those I've never met, asking for more discussion on the everyday practical issues of doing ministry with and for older adults has led to writing this book. There is a great need for discussion by pastors, lay persons, professional care givers and family members.

The following pages rely heavily on some of these articles which have appeared in *The* **Vision**. The articles used in this book are highlighted. Writing them over the last eleven years has helped me clarify my theology of care and helped me sharpen the focus of my ministry with older adults. It is frustrating, challenging and fun all at the same time. Most importantly, to my great astonishment, it has deepened my faith. I have seen the teachings of the Church played out in the lives of the older adults. I trust the pages to follow will lead you to love the ministry with older adults and the caring for them as much as I do.

Jim Stinson

NOTE: The stories told in the following pages are all factually correct. In most instances the names have been changed for the sake of protecting the privacy of the individuals.

INTRODUCTION:
A New Attitude

Stories are wonderful and wonder filled. They can make you laugh. They can make you cry. They can make you reexamine who you are. They can teach you a better way to live life. In the aftermath of the terrible tragedy in Sandy Hook, Ct, and other such horrible massacres there are questions that yearn for answers that will not come. I find myself remembering a story from the Native American tradition. In fact I heard it again in a sermon right after the massacre. It speaks to the question of how and why to go forward in the face of such unspeakable tragedy; in the face of evil. And it speaks to an approach to caring for the aging.

A young girl asks her grandmother the question.

"Grandmother, why do people hurt other people?

"My dear, every person has two wolves living within them. One is a good wolf that seeks to lead the person in the right direction. The other is a bad wolf that seeks to lead the person in a bad direction. These two wolves fight constantly with each other."

"But Grandmother, which wolf wins?"

"The one you feed, dear child, the one you feed!

In every instance we would do well to remember to feed the good wolf; which is to say, to feed the promptings of God within us.

The thought occurs that this story applies to our caring for and ministering to older adults on several levels. The changes that come with aging often lead to a sense of helplessness and despair; to doubting there are ways to get through tough days. Often the wrong wolf; the wolf of despair and helplessness is fed. What a gift it is when we bring older adults in crisis to hear this story and its ramifications for seeing their lives differently.

We may never have answers that satisfy them. We may never understand why their bodies and minds so often fail them. We may never fully understand the losses they experience. We may never really get how difficult it sometimes is to navigate aging. But as people of faith, we affirm a God who loves us. We know the words of Jesus as he speaks to all peoples; *"Come to me and I will give you rest."* We know that the promise is for all people regardless of age or circumstance. We know to find that rest, to find peace filled living we have to pay attention to the common call to feed the wolf of hope and promise.

We know that this call is not always easy to follow, especially when afflicted by the 'ravages' of aging. It is difficult to call people to hear the call as they age. It is especially so when they are aging in a culture that does not fully value them. It is a time when so many, including the aging themselves, hear the words 'old' and 'aging' and hear negatives. To be about the work of caring for our older family members, friends, and parishioners, we need to first reclaim the words 'old' and 'aging.' There is nothing inherently negative about either word. It is learned attitudes and biases that shape our response to them. Two very different attitudes are heard in words I hear nearly every day in my work as Director of Spiritual Life for United Methodist Homes. I hear people expressing joy and fulfillment in the midst of the 'travails' of aging. One of residents said it best recently. "Despite the difficulties that go with it, I am having the time of my life!" Conversely I hear people complaining about their lives every day. Yet another resident capturing the negative view said recently: "There is nothing positive about aging and being old."

So what leads to either attitude? Fortunately my position has given me a laboratory to explore answers for this question. The average age of residents at UMH is well up into the late eighties and early nineties. The last eleven years in my full-time 'retirement' position have convinced me that caring for, and ministering to the aging, is about helping people find the reasons to see 'old' and 'aging' as positives. The question is how to accomplish that task? How do we provide the vision to see all of life – even the process of aging – as a gift to be lived fully and joyfully? T. S. Eliot, in his *The Love Song of J. Alfred Prufrock,* uses a phrase that has stuck with me since college days when I first read the poem. Among other things, the poem has J. Alfrock Prufrock musing about the meaning and worth of his life. When first reading it, as a naïve, star struck, young man, bursting with enthusiasm and energy, certain I could make a real difference in the world, it appeared too morose. I wanted to scream at the questions Eliot raised. I did not have to wonder about life's meaning or purpose. Of course it was worthwhile and significant. I hear it differently now. Time has moved me to a fuller picture of life which, needless to say, is not all roses. Maturing and aging has led to a new appreciation of the lines which affected this young collegian: *and would it have been worthwhile, after the sunsets and the dooryards and the sprinkled streets…would it have been worthwhile?* At seventy plus, the world looks different than at nineteen. Experience has taught me that life always presents us with circumstances that prompt the question. Indeed older adults often spend a considerable amount of time examining their lives, asking questions of meaning and relevance, asking in their own way: *after all would it have been worthwhile?*

In fact, it is such a common experience that a new vocabulary has arisen to describe the phenomenon. It is Life Review. Knowing how common asking such questions is has sparked a field of activity; a field that encourages older adults to reminisce, to review the events of their lives in a more structured way. The purpose of such activity is to create an environment is which the one reviewing her life discovers the wisdom gained over a lifetime and discovers the strength and the power to move beyond the questions. The older adult discovers there is meaning even if questions remain unanswered. For the person sees in Life Review that he has what it takes to live in the present moment just as he had what it took to live in other moments of his life.

Ministry with, caring for older adults, begins with creating environments in which review is welcomed and shared. It happens in settings where reminiscing is welcomed; where repeating stories of the past are seen as moments of enlightenment, rather than as "just another story I've heard a hundred times before." It blossoms when people are allowed to ask the difficult questions posed by Eliot. Only in asking can answers be heard.

I grow old, I grow old.

I shall wear my trousers rolled.

Rather than bemoaning the image conjured up in these lines from Eliot, the task of caring for older adults is to recognize the realities of the aging process, allowing the questions to be asked, and in so doing allowing a discovery of life's meaning even in the face of the questions.

Where do we begin? How we do approach caring for the aging? We begin with the basics. How do we understand the task? We begin with clarity, using words and ideas that all can hear and understand. Hence the following section regarding language.

SPIRITUALITY AND WHOLENESS
(A new language)

The idea for this book began in 2002 when I officially retired as a United Methodist minister from the New York Annual Conference. The reason for retiring at sixty years of age was the offer of the position as Director of Spiritual Life for United Methodist Homes, Inc. Having been a pastor for nearly forty years at the time, I was ready for a new adventure. It has been an adventure in learning and growing ever since. As one might expect, the first step was to figure out what it meant to be Director of Spiritual Life. Particularly it was to figure out what the title implied, in terms of serving a not for profit agency, whose mission is the care and housing of older adults in multiple settings. UMH owns and operates a full retirement community in Shelton, CT. This community includes a skilled nursing and rehabilitation center and two assisted living communities and cottages for largely independent seniors. In addition, it owns and operates two additional communities in CT, as well as one in Memphis, Tennessee.

While covenanting with the United Methodist Church to adhere to practice and language consistent with the denominations policy and beliefs, the population and staff of UMH represents a wide spectrum of faith communities, as well as those of organized faith. The task was to discover and learn ways to be faithful to this covenant, as well as to my own specific understanding of what it means to be a faithful servant of the United Methodist Church, while remaining open and helpful to such a diverse community. The understanding grew within me was to do so would require a 'new language.' All of my life has been informed by 'church language,' language used by a faith institution to guide its people in the art of being 'Christian, (another word which needed new language in my new role.) So the task of developing a language to fit the situation, without compromising core values and beliefs, began.

The first step was to use the word 'spirituality' more often than the words 'religion' and 'faith.' It became very clear that not to do so would quickly close down open dialogue with those who saw life and faith differently than I did. That would include some residents and staff. There is a broader agreement, generally speaking, among people about the meaning of the word spiritual than there seems to be about religion and faith. All people on some level are naturally spiritual, meaning all people search for meaning in their lives. All people, consciously or otherwise, want to know their lives make sense and to have value. Spirituality in this sense is a part of who we are. Some are more aware than others of this fact. Indeed institutional religions provide a path for nurturing and growing one's spirituality. With few exceptions, people seek a connection with others, with the world around them, and with their own understanding of God or the Sacred. Spirituality is the desire to connect with the sacred with a sense of reverence, respect and awe, which not incidentally is part of the root meaning of the Latin word *religio*. The awareness of this has made a difference in the search for a new language and has given me a handle on how to go about being Director of Spiritual Life, without violating my personal faith. What is essential to my attempt to walk faithfully through life is to know a way to be spiritual on the deepest level, to know how to connect with God, with others, with the world and with myself. Putting aside 'church language' is appropriate to a diverse population. It does not violate anything I hold to be true. The 'church language' is still very much a part of my ministry, but it is reserved for situations where people speak 'my language,' most especially Christian worship services and settings, as well as when working with someone who 'speaks this language. It is important for anyone caring for someone who does not share the same language of faith to be aware of the distinction being made, people of any age group, including older adults, come from many different vantage points, even within the same faith tradition. To dialogue with them about important issues in their lives requires that we use language they understand.

Another step in the journey has been to explore the implications of ministering effectively as this understanding of a common spirituality continued to unfold. So much has been written in recent years in this subject. One aspect of this common spirituality is the mind- body – spirit connection and its meaning for a 'whole' or 'well' person. This is not unknown in traditional faith communities. In fact it resonates quite well with basic Christian thought, which teaches that following a spiritual path leads to wholeness or salvation of mind, body and spirit. It is intriguing that the word salvation (a key word to Christians of every stripe) has the root meaning of wholeness. No matter what else it means to any specific Christian, the promise of salvation, the call to a fuller life, is a call to wholeness, a call to pay attention to mind, body and spirit so that wholeness may be experienced.

It is easy to talk about salvation (a word loaded with layers of meaning within the Christian faith system) in terms of wholeness (a term less loaded). The goal of ministry with an older person, as with any person of any age, is to open the possibility for finding this wholeness. It is, to use another word, to open the possibility for healing. Healing is yet another word that must be parsed. In 'church language' it is often used interchangeably with cure. I have been frequently asked as a pastor to pray for healing. What the person asking for such prayer usually means is will I pray for a cure? Cure means that whatever is ailing a person will somehow disappear. Maybe that happens for some, but the reality is that it does not happen for most. Healing, however, is more properly a spiritual event. It happens when a person finds the connections we have discussed and feels whole and at peace despite the physical reality. This can happen to anyone! This does happen often!

I will always remember Betty. She entered my life one day when the Brooklyn Methodist Hospital called and asked if I would visit her. The caller explained that Betty lived around the corner from me and might benefit from a pastoral visit. "Sure," I said, "but can you tell me anything about her and why I might be helpful? The story was told of a woman who had become a frequent visitor to the Emergency Room. She came with all sorts of ailments, none of which seemed to have any medical reason to exist. "In fact," said the caller, "all the tests have come back negative. The problem is that she refuses our efforts to see a counselor which we would provide, if she were willing." Then she said something startling to this (at the time) very young, inexperienced pastor. "Clearly she has a spiritual issue. That's your domain." Long before knowing anything more inclusive about the word spirituality, it began to take on a clearer and deeper meaning for me. Unknowingly I was entering into a new understanding of what healing and wholeness and their relationship to salvation was all about.

I made an appointment with Betty for the next day, not even sure if or why she agreed to let me visit. But she did! Her story was simple, but complicated. He husband had died a few months earlier in a city hospital. When it was clear that he was not going to survive, she made it very clear that the staff was to notify only her when he died. Under no circumstances were they to contact her stepsons, from whom she and her husband had been estranged since their marriage. Upon hearing of his death she made arrangements for a cremation. There were no obituaries nor was there a service of remembrance. She kept his ashes in her bedroom and simply went forward with her life. She had no support during this time from anyone. Through her own actions, she had become disconnected from everyone, even the one connection that had given her life meaning. In other words, she was spiritually ill. She lacked wholeness, without any vehicle for finding it again.

With her permission, the following day she and I shared a time of remembrance in her living room. We talked about Bill. We talked about their life together. We shared prayers together. Most importantly of all we talked about the power of forgiveness to heal brokenness to restore wholeness. It did not take her long to realize that she would never heal without making new connections, without new sources of support.

Betty's entrance into my life was powerful! Especially when she began to regularly attend the church I was serving. "Because," she said, "I know I need God and God's people if I am ever going to feel whole again."

How much better an explanation of the mind-body-spirit connection can there be? Betty quickly lost her symptoms, quickly stopped her visits to the Emergency Room. She had begun to heal! She had begun to experience wholeness because she was able to connect with the God she understood, with people in a wider community and with herself. A healthy spirituality does that for people! 'Church language' may have helped her because at one time in her life that was her language. The language of 'spirituality' also does that.

In ministering to and in caring for older adults language makes a difference between effective and ineffective care. The previous sections on a new attitude and this one on spirituality and wholeness and wellness are the basis for all that follows.

For Further Thought

Have you ever traveled to a foreign country where you did not understand the native language? Have you ever tried to ask for directions in that country? You may have heard a word here or there that was familiar, but even so missed the important details. Can you remember the frustration? Was there any part of you that wanted to say, "Why can't you simply speak my language?"

People from different religious traditions might feel the same way when we talk to them in our own religious language, guessing at the meaning of our words, understanding a word here or there. People who have no formal religious tradition may not understand anything that is being said. The author suggests that the one seeking to care for someone has an obligation to learn the other person's language for meaningful dialogue to flow. Do you agree? Why? Why not?

What are some of the ways you might try to learn a new language? What language would you be willing to change? What language would you be unwilling to change? What would the criteria for changing language be?

SEEING THE
WHOLE PERSON

One of the earlier articles I wrote was titled I HATE BINGO! I LOVE BINGO! In it I noted how different my attitude toward retirement is than my brother's. Like me, he is an ordained United Methodist pastor. He is only fifteen months younger than I am and therefore is facing the aging process as well. He is enjoying a part time retirement, having worked all his life and is ready to "relax and enjoy." On the other hand, although officially retired, I have no desire to stop doing what I'm doing and still work fulltime. Neither attitude is necessarily better than the other. But they are different! In that same article I talked about Muriel and Mike, residents at our Wicke Health Center. "I hate Bingo. It's an idiotic game. I wish they would stop asking me to play. I'd rather read a book" is Muriel's position. Mike however says, "I'd wish they would play Bingo every day of the week."

The question for people seeking to be with and helpful to older adults is: "What gives? Don't all people age the same way? Don't they all have the same needs? Even though we know the answer to these questions, we often act as if we do not. We act as if all people age the same way, as if all old people have the same needs, the same likes, the same dislikes. Some of the responses to this particular article speak of this phenomenon.

> *"How do you come up with different ideas about the same topic so often?"*

> *"I never stopped to think that there was so much involved in doing ministry with and for older adults."*

> *"I often forget 'older adults' is a catchall category. As with all people, older adults do not fit neatly into a category, They are all unique.*

I come up with different ideas about the same topic so often because no two people are alike, not even as they age. There is so much variety among older adults that no single approach to doing ministry with them is sufficient. Just as we have learned that effective ministry with teenagers begins with listening, with hearing their perceived needs and desires and responding accordingly, we need to find ways to effectively minister with older adults. We need to learn to listen, allowing them to lead us rather than the other way around. We need to know their individual needs, their likes and dislikes. We need to find a way to leave our assumptions behind and truly listen and shape ministry accordingly.

It was this effort that prompted the following thoughts.

"I don't know why God has allowed me to live this long. I'm of no use to anyone."

I cannot guess how many times I've heard this sentiment expressed. The "Lone Ranger" in me reflexively wants to ride in on my white horse and rescue the one caught in such a sad, lonely state. But the other side of me knows that nothing I say or do will change how the person feels. All people - including older adults - have a right to feel what they feel and a need to safely express what they feel.

How then do I respond? How can I effectively witness to a faith that finds value in every moment, in every stage of life? I can listen! I can encourage further conversation exploring the person's life story, allowing that person to discover his/her own reason to be alive. One response our Wesley Village Community (United Methodist Homes) in Shelton, CT has been making to this all too common feeling is the Vital Life Stories Program. In it, volunteers are trained to carefully and intentionally solicit a resident's life story, writing only what the person offers. The story is then read to the resident who edits it for clarity of meaning.. Amazingly as they tell their stories they begin to light up as they discover how full, how meaningful their lives have been so far. When the story is complete the volunteers are trained to ask: "What do you think the next chapter of your story might say?" Invariably in telling their stories, they recognize how relationships have played a role in their lives and how they continue to do so. More often than not, residents who began by saying they had nothing to say, having outlived their usefulness, discover that if they can identify important relationships in their current situation, that they feel better.

This comes as no surprise to Christians, does it? Relationships define us and give us meaning. Offer those feeling as if their lives are over an opportunity to see the relationships. The Spirit will do the rest!"

We cannot witness to the Gospel's message that God loves every individual for her own particularity, for his own uniqueness, until and unless we enter into that particularity, that uniqueness. Ministry with and for older adults begins with listening. Anything less risks falling into assumptions that may or may not be true and which may damage the person with its hidden message "you're all the same." Jesus, we remember, asked a most important question of the one seeking his healing touch, "What do you want me to do for you." A ministry of healing does well to begin with the same question. We are most helpful when we are being led by the ones for whom we are caring. It is only as we know a person that we can begin to know the need of that person. It is only as the person knows her need, that the Christian witness of hope can be heard and accepted.

It is important though to know more than a person's limitations or history. We need to know a person's attitude and approach to life. This does not come without careful listening and without building a trusting relationship. It is work! But without doing the work, it is too easy to see an older adult as less than whole, as less capable of dealing with life's issues. Because a person is physically limited or a bit slower than in younger years does not mean he should be cut off from the reality of life, from its ups and downs. In my listening to older adults, I've heard them say, "My children do not listen to me. They treat me like a child! They try to tell me what to do and what not to do.

How often I have heard older adults complain that their family members keep information from them! How often I have seen them diminished by those who love them as they assume Mom or Dad "cannot handle" this or that piece of "bad news." These are the loved ones who unintentionally see their parents, grandparents, and family members only in terms of their limitations. It is this aspect of not seeing a whole person that led me to write "Sharing Bad News with the Older Adult." It was written in response to a situation involving a parent of a friend of mine.

Her grandson is seriously ill, possibly even terminally ill, but the family hasn't said anything to her. The consensus is that 'Grandma' has enough problems of her own to worry about. 'Why make her feel bad about something she cannot change?' How often in the name of compassion, we hide the truth from the aging! Both lay persons and clergy often take this route of dealing with difficult issues.

My question to them is always the same. How would you feel if your family arbitrarily left you out of such a situation? How would you feel to know nothing about a family members' illness and suddenly be told that person has died? An older adult, generally speaking, regardless of his physical condition, has not lost the ability to care, to feel, to show compassion. To deny a person that privilege is to tell her what she may already fear, that she really is no longer important. To not tell the person about such things is to set up a dynamic of mistrust. Why would she believe you the next time that she asks about a family member or friend if you have already lied to her before? Unless there is an overwhelming psychological or physical reason for keeping the truth from the older adult, he has the right to be informed.

How that information is shared is important! Who will be there to assist in the processing of the information? Who will support the person in the days to come as 'coming to grips' sets in?

Attitude matters! Is the one relaying the information comfortable with someone else's emotions? Can they allow any feelings to be okay? Do they understand sickness and death to be part of the natural process of life, allowing them peacefulness in sharing the news?

Spirituality matters! Is the one sharing the news ready to see physical issues as only part of the story, able to allow the older adult to share his faith (or lack of it) without critique? Is he or she comfortable with prayer if that is what the older adult wants at such a time?

If you believe, as I do, that aging is often over-emphasized at the expense of seeing a whole person, you will resonate with my reasoning. Being older does not make a person less capable of handling the difficult moments of life. In fact it may enhance the ability. There is wisdom that comes with aging. Older adults have spent a lifetime learning how to deal with the truth. Trust them with it! Quite possibly they will teach you something about dealing with difficult times!

This article elicited some interesting responses. Several senior citizens who had serious physical limitations wrote to thank me for giving them something to share with their family members. Obviously they understood experientially what I was saying. Some people who were 'caring for an aging family member' had a more difficult time with what I said. "If I tell her the bad things, won't it make her depressed? Won't I make a tough situation worse since she knows she can't do anything about the situation anyhow? Won't sharing tough news with her diminish her hope?"

The truth which I observe almost daily is that older people, unless they are seriously impaired cognitively, have a large capacity for coping with the truth, a capacity developed over a life time of dealing with all manner of events. And this capacity extends even to those times when the difficult news involves them. I have often been asked to not tell a person of his or her condition. I have always resisted that request. I have always counseled family members and friends to trust the power of their relationship and to trust the ability of an older person to handle the truth. My experience is that when honesty prevails the older adult is often able to lead the rest of the family and circle of friends toward acceptance. This experience led to the following article called "Witnessing to Hope When Visiting and Caring for Older Adults." I believe the attitude suggested applies whether the person is at home or with a family member or in an institutional setting.

I read in Richard Morgan's book, No Wrinkles on the Soul,(Upper Room Books, Nashville,1990) that 'years wrinkle the skin, but to give up hope wrinkles the soul.' As I shave each morning it is quite evident that the first part of the statement is true. As I visit with the residents and patients at Wesley Village I have come to know the second half is true also. We cannot do much about the wrinkled skin (Botox not withstanding) but we can do something about wrinkled souls.

Tragically I too often visit those who have come to believe that aging is only about sickness and dying, whose family and friends and church have done little, if anything, to counter the claim. They are the folk who seem to sit and wait and who have come to see life as a burden to be laid down. As a result they are unhappy, dispirited wrinkled souls.

When visiting older adults in their homes, in the hospitals or nursing homes, it is often difficult to know what to say that will not sound trite or condescending. It is difficult to 'confront' the aging with another vision - the vision that life always has possibility and opportunity. It is not always what a 'wrinkled soul' wants to hear. But it is an integral part of the Christian message. We are called to bear witness to this vision nonetheless. How then do we do so?

"A few suggestions follow! There are things to do and things not to do! But the one visiting needs to use inner resources in deciding how to do so. These are ideas that work for me.

1. *Affirm the person and the feelings! 'I've never experienced that! Would you care to tell me more about it?' Never say something like, 'You are a Christian, you know better than that.'*
2. *Redirect the negatives! 'Yet here you are. You must have amazing resources and internal strength to have gotten this far. How did*

you do it?' Get the person to willingly reflect on her/his ability, rather than inability.

3. *Affirm the positives! 'I'm not sure you agree with me, but it seems as if God has given you the strength you need to cope.'*

4. *Point toward the possibilities! "Does anyone not get visitors every day? I wonder if they would like a short visit from you?" "I remember how much you like to read. Did you know there's a weekly book club in this building?" Simple observations on your part can raise the consciousness of new possibilities*

5. *Be a witness to hope by demonstrating that you expect more from the one you visit, always bearing in mind real limitations, physically, mentally and spiritually.*

6. *Avoid offering false hope! "You'll get better and be back to normal soon. Just hang in there." The truth may be very different and you and the person you are visiting likely already know it.*

7. *Visit ready to listen and learn! The older adult will sense that and be more willing to share with you."*

These approaches send a clear message to the older adult. "I value what you feel and say." "I don't always know what you are facing but I do sense your ability to deal with it." "I am willing to accompany you on your journey." They open the possibility of that person revealing herself to you and allowing ministry to happen. Most importantly they allow that person to be seen as more than a disease or a frailty or an aging body. They allow a whole person to be seen.

The gospel promise of salvation, which is the essence of Christian ministry, is a promise of healing and wholeness. When someone is called to salvation he is called to abundant life, something she may feel missing as age takes its toll. Who better to deliver this message than someone who is convinced that God seeks to keep the promise for each individual? Who better than someone convinced that age is not a criteria for experiencing the fulfillment of this promise? Who better than one who knows the healing power of God? As those who would be in ministry with older adults, our goal is to enable this fulfillment to be claimed by the ones for whom we care.

I am careful here to note that a ministry of healing is not the same as a ministry of curing. Curing is about ending a specific illness or condition, something which usually does not happen for the aging. Ultimately we die and it is usually from some illness or condition. Healing is about *being* able to live fully in the moment, (not necessarily being free of ailments), feeling connected to God and the world. This belief led to the following article.

"Wellness!" Have you noticed how this word has entered our vocabulary in a big way? It is ill defined and used in a variety of ways. Gyms use it to lure new customers, promising feelings of new vitality and better health. Hospitals use it to promote community outreach programs, suggesting that certain regimens will help forestall the need for hospitalizations. Long-term care facilities use it to encourage residents to stay in the best physical shape they can, despite their limitations. And on the list goes.

My favorite understanding of "wellness" centers on the biblical understanding of "salvation." It suggests a sense of peace that comes from being at one with God and one's neighbor. It suggests not just a release from sin, but an integration of the whole person, of mind, body and spirit. "Salvation" and "wholeness" are basically the same word in Greek. Wellness, it seems to me, has to do with knowing salvation, with knowing that mind, body and spirit are working together to reveal the saving presence of God within us. As our wedding ceremonies say: I will love you in sickness and in health," so too does God's salvation make the same promise. Being physically well is not enough! Being mentally well is not enough! Being spiritually well is not enough! We need to keep all three aspects in the best condition possible, even knowing the body and the mind will likely falter one day.

But what a disservice we do when we allow any of the three to be seen separately. If we care for the mind, reading, studying, doing puzzles and such, and do not care for the body and spirit, we are only offering a part of salvation. Likewise if we care for the body, neglecting the other two, we are only offering a portion of what we have to offer. And if we care only for the spirit, praying, worshipping, reading devotional pamphlets, we are missing part of the equation.

In doing ministry with older adults, it is all too easy to forget this understanding of salvation and to deal only with the physical, if the person is ill or frail. It is too easy to neglect the physical and the spiritual, if the person's mind is failing. It is too easy to deal only with the spiritual (often meaning the 'church stuff' - praying, reading scripture, etc.) when mind and body are less than what they once were. Churches and any group seeking to offer salvation in this context will do well to struggle with how to offer ministry that addresses the whole person - body, mind and spirit.

How to do so is an ongoing question that deserves our time and attention.

In short the Gospel compels us to offer a ministry of salvation. Older adults are no less in need of this ministry than anyone else. They too are healed when touched by a love that dares to see a whole person (the hopes and the fears, the dreams and the nightmares) touched by a love that will walk with them every step of the way. The Gospel compels us to enter a ministry of presence. If we are going to minister to a whole person we will need to be there in body, mind and spirit if we ever hope to offer salvation to others. This is time consuming. It involves a willingness to see and know a whole person, involves having an awareness of our own salvation. This is an awesome task, but one that adds to our wholeness, even as it helps another.

For Further Thought

What are the elements of good listening? When have you experienced being truly listened to? What can you replicate from this experience in relating to others?

What experience have you had of giving someone bad news? What have you learned that could help older adults and those who love them?

When have you been left out of important decisions? How did this omission make you feel? Did you reassert yourself in the network of decision makers? If so how? What hints might you glean from this that would serve older adults?

This section speaks of the importance of the "Vital Life Stories" program. When is remembering the past an opportunity for deepened relationships and when does it inhibit an older adult from engaging meaningfully in the present day?

Are you comfortable speaking with older adults about their spirituality? Do you agree that "Spirituality matters?" If so, what do you imagine will be the opportunities and pitfalls in talking about spirituality with older adults?

MINISTERING TO THE WHOLE PERSON

If indeed the task of ministry with and for older adults is to call them into wholeness despite their situations (just as it is the goal of ministry with anyone), how do we do so? Especially how do we do so within a cultural context that runs from age as if it were a disease to be avoided at all costs, a context that often treats the aging as if they were children needing to be cared for, a context that denies the mortality that it seeks to hide? As already suggested one of the concerns which is vitally important and which too often gets short shrift is honesty. In the name of compassion we often keep the truth from them. "The news would only upset Mom." "Dad would not know what to do with the bad news, it would only depress him." These are the things we tell ourselves and others as reasons for our lack of honesty. Is it not possible they say more about our own unwillingness or inability to deal with the truth? Are these statements about us rather than about the aging person who, simply by his advanced years, bears witness to an ability to deal with the realities of life? The following two articles sought to raise these questions with those ministering to such people, both family members and others.

Some years ago my father-in-law was struggling with terminal illness. My mother-in-law had decreed that no one was to tell him the truth about his condition. She did not "want him to lose hope." My wife and I had a difficult time with that decision and struggled as to how to respond. Did we respect my mother-in-law's decision, or did we, as our hearts told us to do, speak the truth?

As we struggled my father-in-law deteriorated. One morning, while visiting him, he was in a particularly weak condition. He looked sick and had no energy. I took a chance, decided to skirt the decision that had been made. I wouldn't, I decided, tell him he was terminally ill. But I would open the door for him to talk about it, if he decided to do so.

"George, how are you feeling today? You look terrible!"

Never will I forget the response. He filled with tears, looked me in the eye, and said, 'Thank you! I know I look terrible! I know I am quite ill and not going to get better. But I was afraid to say so. I thought it would upset everyone.' We spent the rest of that morning talking and listening as George shared his wishes for his last days and his wishes for his funeral. With his permission I waited for my mother-in-law to get home and sent for my wife. When they were both there, I asked George to share his thoughts with them.

His last months were filled with honest sharing with those he most loved. They shared with him; he shared with them. It was a beautiful time for the relationships to flourish in a new way.

I relearned a lesson that day. It has deeply affected the way I visit the terminally ill. I still do not tell them 'what I know.' That is, unless asked by family or doctor to do so. But I do open the door for honesty. I ask questions! How are things going? Is the doctor giving you any new information? Do you want to share what is going on inside of you? Hopefully I do so only if I sense that our relationship allows those kinds of probing questions. And hopefully I ask in such a way that an unwillingness or inability to share or do so at that moment is graciously accepted.

The lesson relearned is that 'the truth does set us free.' Only when we are able to acknowledge our situation are we able to open ourselves to the presence of a loving God, who walks with us in every moment of our lives. Only when we are honest can we discover that terminal *illness is not necessarily the enemy. The enemy is living as if we have to face it quietly, stoically and alone.*

When visiting a terminally ill person, old or young, respect them enough to create an atmosphere of honesty. Respect them enough to allow them to talk about their situation at their own pace and their own comfort level."

The responses were varied. Many voiced instant agreement and asked how to be honest after years of hearing others tell them that to do so would be harmful. Others were worried responses that it might be bad advice that would do damage. To the former there is no need to respond. To the latter I respond with their question. Suppose not telling the person the truth is doing damage? The entire hospice movement bears testimony that people not only can accept the truth, but that they live as full lives as possible right up until they die once they do accept it. There is no doubt in my mind that 'the truth does set us free.' Denying someone the privilege and the healing that comes with that acceptance lessens the chances of fully knowing the promise of the Gospel - the promise of salvation, of wholeness and the ensuing peace that brings.

The danger in this article was that people might hear the lesson of the need for honesty with the terminally ill and not hear it in every other aspect of ministering with and to the older adult. Do we discuss dementia and Alzheimer's disease with those who have them? Do we allow inappropriate behavior from our aging loved ones, our church members, or others with whom we minister, excusing the behavior because they are old? Or do we expect the same rules of behavior be observed by everyone? Unless there are cognitive reasons for a person being unable to live by accepted standards of behavior, we do a disservice if we 'let her off the hook.' What we are really saying when we do so is "You are not really 'like us, you are 'different.' This is a fear of too many seniors already! The gospel calls young and old, healthy and infirm, to the same standards of loving, responsible relationships. Our ministry needs to emphasize this at every age level.

If we are to witness to the wholeness that is possible we must be honest. If an older person insults us, or anyone, that person needs to be held accountable. If she has no friends because of her behavior, it is an act of love and ministry to share that with her. If he is feeling isolated and alone because he will not take steps to change that feeling, it is an act of love and ministry to share that with him. Honesty, offered in love and empathy for the person, is the key to effectively engaging the older adult in this important discussion! We neglect it at a price. Salvation in the terms we have been talking is at stake! This is true in every situation! Are there times when withholding information is the right approach? Perhaps! But they are few and far between. If we are going to honor an older person as a complete human being, there is no reason to lie, dissemble or withhold information. To do so is to diminish that person. Hence the following!

What do I say to my mother? The doctor says she has Alzheimer's and increasing dementia. He also says that, for her own safety, she needs to be in a supervised setting. If I tell her she has to move, she'll tell me to mind my own business. She can make her own decisions. If I tell her the medical reasons for having to move, she'll get angry and deny there is anything wrong, even though the signs of a problem have been evident for quite some time.

With these words began a conversation and ultimately a meeting with her mother that was quite painful. The daughter rightly predicted her mother's response. It was most difficult to be part of that conversation, knowing how frightened and hurt each person was. It fortunately ended better than expected. The mother was admitted to the hospital with an infection (which she knew she had) and while there was monitored and had her medications carefully watched. She and her daughter agreed on a new home setting for her. It doesn't always work out as well! It sometimes takes more than one discussion. But putting it off only makes it more difficult. No matter how painful, the truth needs to be shared.

The incident caused me to look again at ways to handle such situations. Some suggested things to consider when called upon to minister in such instances are:

1. *Honesty is still the best policy. People have a right to know their situation to the best of their ability to understand.*
2. *Recognize that anger, hopelessness, despair often cause people to say hurtful things to the ones they love the most. Do not argue with your loved one.*
3. *If you must argue, argue with the disease, not the one afflicted.*
4. *Keep sight of how you would feel if someone delivered such news to you.*
5. *Bring a neutral third party with you for support, as well as for opening the possibility that another voice, other than a loved one's might be heard more objectively.*
6. *Both by word and actions reassure the person of God's presence and love, even in this situation.*
7. *Affirm your awareness that this is a lonely road to travel and that you will travel it with your loved one.*

It is never easy to face and to share such news, but who better to do so than a loved one?

However it is easier if the one in need of assistance knows that he is being listened to and valued. This is so basic that I find it hard to understand why so many caregivers miss it. Even more so I find it incredible that ministers, lay ministers, and others who care about the aging find it so difficult to listen. How often I shudder when I observe some of these people dispensing advice - "You need to do this, it's for your own good" kind of advice - seemingly dismissing the feelings, perceptions, fears and such of the older adult as immaterial. No wonder most of the responses to the following came from older people, one of whom seemed to sum up all the other responses. "Right on," she said. "I cut out your article and gave it to my daughter who needed to read it."

"My Dad doesn't know how to listen. He doesn't ask what I think or feel, he just tells me what to do." Any of us who have ever worked with teens know how often this complaint is heard. That's not a problem

just for teens, it's a problem at any age. No one likes to be told what to do.

Some time ago a resident at Wesley Village was sharing her concerns about her relationship with her daughter. "I get so frustrated and angry with her. She is always telling me what to do."

> *"Mother, you should have your hair done every week!"*

> *"Mother, you need to eat more greens!"*

> *"Mother, you have to get involved in more of the activities that are offered!"*

> *"Mother, this!"*

> *"Mother, that!"*

"I wish just once she would stop telling me what to do and simply sit and listen to me. Maybe then she would understand why I do what I do and why I feel what I feel."

She got me to wondering how often, with good intentions, we presume to know what older adults want and need. How often we assume we know how they feel. We plan events for them in our churches and never include them in the planning. We offer advice freely, unconsciously perhaps, assuming they don't know what they want or need to do. We minister to them and for them, which assumes they are incapable of being in ministry with us.

A retired minister in our community, in his late nineties, carries on an active ministry and presence among us. Recently, I asked him if he wanted to be relieved of some of his "duties," only to be told he would let me know when and if that became the case. I needed to hear him and let him set the pace, rather than my own assumptions about what was good for him and what wasn't.

With all people, especially older adults, listening is the key ingredient of ministering. Unless cognitively impaired in a serious way, their thoughts, feelings and needs must inform us before we deign to offer advice, programs or any other form of ministry to them.

James Andrew Stinson

Wondering what to do about older adult ministry? Begin with a heavy dose of listening!

Until and unless we internalize these standards, (1) being honest with the older adult and (2) carefully listening to him we will likely continue to do less than offer the gospel. The Scripture presents a picture of Jesus who knows how to listen and who is honest with everyone. Jesus does not quibble in calling sin by its name, he does not hesitate to direct his followers to look at themselves and ask honest questions.

"Who do you say that I am?"

"Your sins are forgiven. Your faith has made you whole."

"Who touched me?"

The stories surrounding these sayings and so many others paint a picture of a Jesus who listened, heard what others were saying, responded without equivocation, and did so with compassion, but nonetheless honesty. We can do no less if we want to present a whole gospel to the older adult.

We cannot offer a gospel of hope to someone with a terminal illness, if we cannot talk with them about the presence of God in such a situation. Ignoring the fact of the illness sets up a relationship where lying and pretending become the norm, hardly conducive to honest witnessing to hope in the midst of despair.

We cannot offer a gospel of resurrected living to someone who clings to the past because it is all he sees as possible. Resurrected living begins with allowing death to the past to take place. Ministry to older adults is often marked by a lack of challenge, by a lack of daring. Older people need to be called to let go of the past - even as we all do - so that they can become free to see the present, with any limitations it might bring, free to live as fully as possible in the moment.

We cannot offer a gospel of forgiveness if we do not listen to the aging, hearing where the hurts, the fears, the faithlessness of the past is still impacting the present. Only when we do so are we able to share the good news that these things are of yesterday, these things are forgiven. Only when we do so are we able to enable the person to face the present moment with love and hopefulness.

If our concern is to offer a gospel of wholeness, we have to find ways to offer hope based in resurrection theology and forgiveness based in grace. The platitudes of "everything will be okay" variety mitigates the possibility of this happening and is yet another way we do not take older adults seriously. When we offer platitudes, it is a sure sign we are not listening. It is a sign of discomfort and avoidance. Ministry with older adults is often a ministry of presence, less about answering questions, more about 'being there.' "Being there" as a loving presence, being open and affirming, setting up a dynamic whereby trust is established and the difficult issues might be addressed.

Also important in ministering to the whole person is being a physical presence as well as a spiritual or religious presence. Central to our faith is incarnation. God took and takes human form, which is to say God is known by physical presence as well as by a spiritual or mystical presence. The old hymn learned in Sunday School years ago still informs my way of doing ministry. "God has no hands but my hands. God has no mouth but my mouth." At least that is how I remember it! Even if I am remembering the words incorrectly, they state clearly and unequivocally the challenge of ministry with anyone, let alone seniors. It is to be the physical presence of the Divine. Quite a challenge! But if it is not accepted, it is quite a loss for those to whom we minister!

How well I remember visiting a parishioner who was dying of AIDS. As I was preparing to leave I asked if there was anything else I could do for him. I still remember his answer. It still sends shivers through my body! "Would you just hold me for a while, no one has done that since I was diagnosed." I sat on the bed and held him as tightly as I could for a 'good long time' as tears streamed down both our faces. As important as this time was for him and for me, his verbal response (matched by a body that had physically relaxed as I held him) has left the deeper impression on me. "Thank you, I already feel better. I was feeling abandoned by everyone, including God. I don't feel that way right now."

Study after study has demonstrated the importance of touching and being touched for the young and the old and the people in between. It still amazes me that the simple act of holding someone restored his sense of God's presence. It amazes me even more that we sometimes forget that in our ministry!

We are called to be the hands of God, are we not?

In this age where we are rightly sensitive to inappropriate touching it is important that we find ways to share a healing touch with those to whom we minister. Especially is this true in ministry to and with older adults. Often they can identify with the dying AIDS patient. Widowed, living alone, away from adult children, their need to be touched is neglected. Other than an occasional handshake or hug they lack for physical touch.

How do we provide that in an appropriate manner?

Here are some suggestions that I use, whenever appropriate. I try hard to be aware of a person's comfort level before using any of these ways.

1. *Holding hands during prayer*
2. *Making the sign of the cross on their foreheads when ending a visit*
3. *Placing my hand on their shoulders as they leave the worship center*
4. *Training visitors in hand massage*
5. *Hugging Using scented oil in a blessing of hands ritual*
6. *Taking their hands as I place the communion bread in it*

Without a physical connection, God may remain a distant reality at best or a non-existent reality at worst. If ministry is to be holistic it must remember the connection between mind, body and spirit. When one is out of sync then so are the other two. Ministry and programs that emphasize one aspect over the other misses the chance to witness to an abundant life on every level.

A word about ministering with and caring for, those who are caregivers is in order. For no one exists in a vacuum. We are all inter-related. If those who are important in our lives are not 'well,' neither are we. If they are not whole, neither are we! We are affected by others. This is especially so in the case of the aging. Their dependence upon others often grows with age and their responses to their lives often reflect the responses of those who care for them. How often, in my work at the United Methodist Homes, I find myself working with family members who are impeding the adjustment of their parent, grandparent, aunt or uncle! It is easy for them to see only the disease and frailty and thus fall into the painful experience of seeing caring for old people as a burden to be borne. It is easy for them to miss the opportunity to see growth for themselves and their loved one in a difficult situation. How easy it is for them to fall into the trap of 'parenting the parent,' with all the energy draining, and spirit sapping such an attitude exacts. It is something to be 'lived through,' rather than something to be experienced. It is something to dread, rather than something to embrace; life-taking, rather than life-giving.

"I'm so tired of being a parent to my parent. It is not natural and it leaves me tired and feeling guilty." Anyone with an aging parent or loved one who is reaching, or has reached, the state of needing assistance with daily routines and medical needs understands this cry.

"My daughter (son) forgets that I'm the parent and makes me so angry when she (he) treats me like a child." Any aging person who needs another person to step in and "do for me what I once did for myself" understands this complaint.

Yet life brings with it times of interdependence and times of dependence! Life brings us to circumstances that require different levels of assistance. All too often these times bring family dynamics to stressful points. The adult child knows the parent needs help! The parent knows help is needed but is resentful when it is provided. Is there a way beyond this reality? Recently a case assessment and case manager who specializes in elder care told me of an insight she received at a training session she attended. She said the speaker suggested that partnering a parent rather than parenting a parent was a better direction, one that too many adult children do not take. I'm not sure of all that might mean! I do know that just the attitude suggested by the word partnering has a soothing effect. It suggests control over one's life is still possible. It suggests that the older adult is still valued for her opinion. It suggests to the older adult that he is not alone in his efforts to deal with the changes in his life and that he still has a say in how to respond to them. It suggests to the adult child that Mom or Dad still want to do the 'parent thing' of making life easier for the child.

There are lots of other implications, some of which I am still pondering. But the change in words speaks volumes about our perception of the aging process. With parenting a parent there is the sense of having one more task added to an already busy schedule. With partnering a parent there is the sense of being creatively involved in a changing, yet on-going relationship.

How helpful it would be if churches would explore this insight with older adults and their children, especially if they did so against the backdrop of the biblical teaching to honor your mother and your father! How helpful it would be if pastors and other care people would be alert to those in their churches who see caring for their aging parents as an added chore rather than an opportunity to deepen a most important relationship!

It is amazing how a change in words can bring new understanding and a change in attitudes! Partnering leads me down a different path than parenting. It feels right, especially as I enter my senior years. For it is how I already know I would want to be treated.

Ministering to the whole person is a challenge, to say the least. But it can also be an incredibly rewarding experience, allowing growth for all involved. It can bring new insights, deeper relationships, deeper faith, and a growing ability to relate in empathy to others. This is especially true in ministering to the whole person as that person ages. We become enriched when we share the final years of a life's journey with someone we love, especially when we do so with careful listening and honesty. In so doing we come to know another person deeper than we ever thought possible, an incredible experience. And the person with whom we share the journey teaches us how to face such a time as we watch them find strength and vision for living their later years.

The reality is that we do not have to have a ministry of questions and answers to be effective. In fact that may be one sure way not to have an effective ministry. When we listen and honestly engage with the older adult he discovers, as do we, that the ability to handle each of life's issues and stages lies within each individual. Christians have many ways of describing this reality. The one that speaks to me is found in the opening pages of Genesis. ***And God created them in God's own image, male and female God created them.*** No matter how we understand this ancient story of creation, its theology is surely one embraced by Jesus. We are created in God's image! We have within us the ability to see as God sees, to hear as God hears, and to experience as God experiences. Allowing a person to "talk it out" with someone who is listening and responding honestly enhances the possibility that person will discover God's vision for her life. There is no way to overstate the need to listen and to be honest if the goal is to witness to a gospel of hope.

For Further Thought

The story of the author and his father-in-law raises the question of honesty. Has anyone, perhaps with good intentions ever lied to you? How did that experience feel? Would you rather have been told the truth? Can you relate to the dilemma posed by the story? Having heard the story, has your mind changed about the importance of telling the truth to an older adult?

Since listening is so important in a caring ministry can you recall a time when you felt you were not being heard? How did that make you feel? Imagine how an older person feels when someone else makes decisions that affect her without being consulted. Is there ever an acceptable excuse for doing so? What might that exception be?

The writer was moved to tears, without words, in his ministry with the AIDS patient. He saw his efforts as effective caring ministry. Words were not sufficient to reach the man. Holding him changed everything. Have you ever not had words to offer that would comfort? What might you have done instead of speaking? How important to older adults in the 'ministry of presence?'

It is said that adult children often become parents to their parents. Has that been your experience, or the experience of someone you know? Would seeking ways to partner with or parent or other older adult offer richer opportunities for the relationship and for the person you care about?

OFFERING A HOLISTIC GOSPEL

Since the goal of ministering with/to older adults is to meet and witness to the whole person, how do we do that? Especially how do we do so when so many grow frail as they age, so many develop physical problems that become time consuming and spirit consuming? There is a reason so many older people spend a good deal of their time talking about illness and death. It is because both are a very present part of their days. It is not always easy to grow old. These natural occurrences play a major role in our aging and often take on a life of their own. Thoughts, attitudes, and faith itself is often changed by this fact. If we are to minister to older adults in their wholeness, we need to move beyond the obvious physical realities before our eyes. If we are to offer a gospel that calls us to abundant living, we have to find ways (without resorting to platitudes) to reclaim the biblical teaching that a person is more than a body. While not talking about the process of aging Paul even so gives us a direction in this regard.

So we do not lose heart. Though our outer nature is wasting away, our inner nature is being renewed every day. For this slight momentary affliction is preparing for us an eternal weight of glory beyond all comparison, because we look not to the things that are seen but the things that are unseen; for the things that are seen are transient, but the things that are unseen are eternal. (2 Corinthians 4:16-18)

For we know that if the earthly tent (body) we live in is destroyed, we have a building (body) from God, a house not made with hands, eternal in the heavens. (2Corinthians 5:1)

Our faith tells us that the body is only part of who we are. Holistic witnessing to that faith to older adults means helping them see beyond the moment. It means that even as we care for their bodies, we find ways to care for their spirits (souls). It does not finally matter how literally we understand these words of Paul. It matters that we appropriate them as the reason for our ministry in the first place. Honesty demands that we affirm that the body will fail and waste away. It is not tragedy or failure when that happens, it is simply the way life moves along. But to say or witness only to that reality is to miss the rest of the Gospel. We are also spirit or soul. It is to that reality we must also minister if we are to attend to the needs of a whole person. Older adults, no less than anyone else and perhaps more than most, must be challenged to see this other truth. As we age and focus more and more on physical needs, that becomes more and more difficult to do. For as we age we bring with us many of our culture's attitudes, including the attitude that sees age largely in terms of disease and weakness. Somehow ministering to a whole person as he ages means calling him back again to his call to follow Jesus into a life lived in love and service. This certainty led to the following.

I've been asked to lead devotions for the seniors that meet in our church. I've never done that before. It is scary, suppose I do it wrong? Do you have any suggestions? I have been amazed at how many phone calls I get from frantic church members asking this and similar questions.

When offered the opportunity to witness to older adults, either in a formal or informal setting, where do we begin? If that is not our question, it ought to be! Witnessing, preaching, sharing our faith, is not something to be done lightly. I think of the numerous times I've been present when such an event took place, and how often I have shuddered at the trivializing of the Gospel that passed for devotion and worship. How often such a time seems to offer banal comments about the afterlife, glib observations about dealing with problems faced by the aging (moving to a new home, death of a spouse, death of friends, for example)! How often such a time, such an opportunity, is met with a poem, a reading about the beauty of nature, rather than a call to commit anew to the challenge and joy of living out the gospel in every circumstance of our lives.

Older adults are no different than anyone else in this regard. We all need to know that Christian living is about becoming, about growing, about reflecting the love of God! We all need to be challenged! We all need to be hearing the truth that while we have breath we have a purpose to live out! How often I have found myself saying to one of our residents in Wesley Village, "What are you doing with the rest of your life? Are you going to let that wheelchair or that walker, or your infirmity, stop you from living as if you know God still loves you and still has a purpose for you?"

When our devotions, our worship does not challenge the older adult, it misses the gospel message that every life is valuable, every life is worth living and, every life has something to offer the world. Unless cognitively unable, every adult can still follow Jesus' mandate to be of service. Every older adult can still be a caring friend to someone in need, can still speak to a lonely neighbor, can still listen to someone else's story. Not to challenge them to become all they can is to suggest that they are no longer needed or valuable, certainly not the message we want to deliver or to which Christians bear witness.

"I've been asked to lead devotions for seniors that meet in our church...do you have any suggestions?"

Yes, I do! Follow the lead of Jesus, remember that all people are called with three simple words, 'Come, follow me!' Plan accordingly and you'll be on the right track.

It seems to me that these observations apply to every form of ministry with older adults. Adult children, pastors, lay ministers, caring committees would enhance their work if they saw older people holistically. They would be more effective in bringing the good news of the gospel if they saw them as Jesus saw them. Jesus did not see through sentimental eyes, or eyes of demeaning pity. He called everyone to live out their awareness of being made in the image of God. He called them to be all that God intended them to be. He called them to glorify their creator even in their suffering. We do a disservice to them if we do anything less!

We are entrusted with a gospel of hope for every circumstance of our lives. It is a gospel that begins with *'Come, follow me!'* It doesn't stop being a call just because we are old. There is a danger that our ministry may become one of doctrine and rules. "To follow Jesus means you must..." kind of witness! I believe Christian ministry with and for anyone at any age is neither doctrinal nor about rules. It is invitational and non coercive. The last thing an older person wants or needs as she maneuvers the path of aging are these things. What she finds helpful and life giving is to experience God's love and to experience God's mercy. Because if she can do that, she can respond with her spirit to the call to: *'Come, follow me!'* Finding ways to open these experiences is the challenge. Undoubtedly there are many ways to do so. But we can be sure they will not take place without a relational component. If we want to lead others to experience God's love and mercy, we need to meet them where they are, rather than where we want them to be. We need to show them a whole person in ourselves, if we want them to find one in themselves. Among other things we must be forthcoming about our fears and lack of answers. "I'm afraid to be in this place. I feel so alone." The typical response from the care giver is condescending and allows the person to feel inadequate. "Don't be afraid! You're not really alone" The statements from the older person, if we listen closely, are often self-revelatory.

"Why do I feel this way? "

"What is wrong with me that I have this fear, no one else seems to?"

It is far better to empathize, to enter the other person's space. "I suspect I would feel the same way if I were in your shoes." Only when we do so is the other person able to hear more encouraging words, able to hear them from someone who 'understands' their viewpoint. It takes time and effort to build that kind of relationship, but is worth it when we see an older person find hope and promise in their later years.

Although I was not thinking of this book when writing the next essay it speaks to what can happen if we see our ministry with older adults in relational terms.

"Jim, will you say the last rites for my mother? The doctor says she will not be alive this time tomorrow morning." "Annette, won't you let me call your Mom's priest to do so? She has always been a faithful member of her church." "No Jim, Mom has told me more than once that when this day came, she wanted me to call you."

What did I do? It was not the first time I had been asked to perform a service for someone from a different religious tradition than mine. I always believed that pastoral care and an ecumenical spirit trumps other considerations. And so the answer was easy. I shared prayers and thoughts about life, death and resurrection with Annette, her Mom and other members of the family.

But these thoughts are not about performing such a service. They are about a lesson I am learning again and again as I do ministry in a long-term care setting where many religious traditions are represented. I'm discovering that most people, as they face life and death questions, want pastoral care, far more than they are concerned about distinctions of church theology. They want to experience the love of God and to be reassured of the wideness of God's mercy. There seems to be the sense that the things that often divide us during our lifetime simply are not important.

Each time I relearn this lesson I recommit to an inclusive ministry. How often lay speakers and clergy are called upon to lead worship in a long-term care facility! How often I hear them forgetting this lesson! We need to be aware of the people to whom we have been called to minister. In nursing homes and such they are Methodists, Episcopalians, Baptists, Roman Catholic and every other possibility. Such a setting requires that we be non-denominational in our approach. It requires that we witness to the good news of Jesus Christ and the overwhelming love of God and trust that God can speak to people through a good pastoral presence. A good sign for me of whether I have done so comes when I hear the comment I heard recently, 'I am not a Methodist but I felt as if I were hearing my own pastor speak to me.'

Christian ministry with the older adult (perhaps with all people) is finally about touching them with the message of God's love and mercy and with helping that experience become a reality for them. It is an exciting ministry that requires openness to all people, a loving heart convinced that Jesus made God visible, committed to sharing that presence with others, and a willingness to remember the message we have heard and to bear witness to it in a way that those for whom going to their 'own' church is not an option will feel as if they are in their 'own' church. It takes time and effort, but well worth both!

A relational ministry erases distinctions that do not matter. Annette was right in asking me to give "the last rites" to her mother. I had a relationship with her Mom, one that was empathetic and had developed a level of trust. If she was able to hear the prayers I shared at the bedside and the words I shared with her family she heard them not as "church prayers and words," but rather as heart-felt from someone who knew her and loved her. Her family heard them the same way and we were able to spend a good bit of time discussing how they would and could move on when their mother, mother-in-law, and grandmother died.

Relational ministry creates situations in which people are free to explore their spirituality freed from the constraints of doctrine and rules. It opens the possibility for the Spirit of God to be sensed and heard in a new way. The Church's doctrine of the Incarnation - the belief that God took human form in Jesus - is an important thing to explore. Its implications are tremendous in our ministry. If God was in Jesus, so too is God in us. This is the clear teaching of Jesus. **"Come, follow me!"** No matter what else that might mean, it surely means that we are called to reveal God in ourselves as well as Jesus. A relational ministry that is self-revelatory and honest is one way to be God's presence for those with whom we minister.

Surely a key to relational ministry with the aging is prayer. The very act itself is relational as it connects the ones praying in a common faith and it connects the ones praying with God. The danger though is the misuse of prayer. It can be used by very caring people as a tool to manipulate the one(s) being prayed for. It can be used to push a theological understanding and subtly suggest that God agrees with that understanding. It can be used to suggest a course of action that the one being prayed for has not decided to follow.

"God help John see your will in all this. Help him to respond in the way we have been discussing."

In fact, John might not believe that God's will has anything to do with his situation. He may not believe that the way that has been discussed is the right way. A better prayer might be "God help us to see ways to respond, ways that might allow us to more nearly do your will." When we pray for others it is good to remember that the Spirit is heard and felt differently by different people. Part of our wholeness is found as we find our own "ears" to hear what God is saying.

Prayer can also be misused if it holds out false promises, or presupposes the result. For Christians the prayer of Jesus contains the guide to prayer's goal. It is to see that '*thy will be done*.' It is important to pray with others, especially those that are sick and hurting, seeking God's strengthening presence as we cope with the circumstances of our lives. It also helps to remember that as important as prayer may be to us, it might not be to others. I will never forget the time a woman (in my first full time appointment) was dying and I visited her in the hospital. As it came time to end the visit I invited her to pray with me. Obviously she felt the invitation was manipulative since she had not indicated a desire to pray with me. Her response to my invitation was clear, not angry, but direct. "If it will make you feel better, go ahead." Since then if I am unsure if sharing a prayer is wanted, I say something like "I have to be going now, please know you will be in my prayers." I have noticed with joy that such a statement often opens the door for the person to say "Will you do so now?"

Some clarifying thoughts on prayer follow!

"Pastor will you pray that my husband be healed?" There are no more troubling words a pastor or any other caring person can hear! For in these words lie volumes of trust and assumptions and hopes. In these words lie expectations that might be unrealistic. The person asking for prayer (young or old) is speaking in short hand of the human experience. Behind these words lie several assumptions. Some of these are:

- *There are some situations in life we cannot handle alone.*
- *God is able and willing to do something about these situations.*
- *The one being asked to pray will be able to get God to respond.*
- *There is strength in the community of faith.*
- *God controls our lives so completely that even life threatening illness is under God's control.*

Theologically I believe all of these things to be true, but the literal interpretation of them needs unpacking. But that is not the point of this article. The point is that there are some events in life that inexorably will lead to death no matter how hard we pray. I believe we are more faithful to the word of Jesus if we constantly distinguish between praying for a healing and praying for a cure. Most people seem to mean pray that I be cured rather than pray that I be healed.

What do I mean? I have been struck by the faith and insight of someone with a life threatening illness that is able to say: "Whether I recover or not, I am going to be okay. God will see to that!" That person, I believe, is healed. Whether a cure occurs or whether it does not, matters less than "the peace that passes all understanding" which is spoken in such an affirmation.

So respond to such requests for prayer carefully and empathetically, helping the person to experience the promise of God, "Lo I am with you always!" Pray for a cure, but pray clearly as well for a healing. And when you do, help the person with whom you are praying to see the difference and to wait on the unfolding of God's love.

So when is prayer an appropriate way of offering the gospel holistically? I don't believe there is a right or wrong answer to the question. It is a matter of being sensitive to the older adult (any person for that matter), rather than your own need or belief. I still remember a professor from seminary who answered this same question one day by saying, "If in doubt, be an answer to prayer rather than saying one." Whether you agree or not is less important than the sentiment. The one to whom we are ministering is the most important person in the room.

Visits to and prayers with older, cognitively impaired, persons need not be frightening. Remember you go as a witness to the God who loves us as we are, is slow to judge and quick to embrace. Go and visit as one who knows that God and, by your loving embracing behavior, let the one being visited know and feel that love.

A goal of ministry with older adults, many of whom no longer feel whole, is to witness to a wholeness that is still there. It is there because we are made in the image of God. That image does not cease to exist because our bodies or minds begin to fail. It may be more difficult to see but it is still there. Circumstances do not change that. When we are witnessing to the wholeness of the person, we are saying something about their sacred worth, a difficult thing to do when working with many older adults, whose bodies or minds seem to belie such a worth. I find insight for doing so in **When I Am An Old Woman I Shall Wear Purple. (ed. Sandra Martz, Papier-Mache, 1987, 2002, 2003))** In it we find this by someone named Joanne Seltzer. It is entitled **Sudden Illness.**

When mother is discharged
from the hospital
you accompany her down
on the same elevator
with a young couple
bringing Baby home.
They call to mind
the Holy Family
until you realize

that every family is holy.
You feel holier-than-thou.

When I read this recently my response was: what a powerful reminder when ministering to/with older adults. How easy it is to forget their holiness, their sacred worth! How easy it is to see frailty, rather than a soul, every bit as valuable to God as when it was housed in a younger, healthier body! How easy it is to become so entangled in the question, "How do I care for this person now?" How easy it is to see the older adult as a project to be cared for, rather than a person to be engaged! We must "realize that every family is holy." Doesn't this imply that every member of every family is holy and sacred, most especially the old and the frail?

What does this mean? How do we affirm the sacred worth of a person, especially as we need to be increasingly concerned about physical care? It is different for each person but certain things are common.

1. An older adult may be less capable than she once was, but her thoughts and wishes still matter.
2. The physical condition does not define the person. It is simply a fact to be acknowledged.
3. The spirit of a person is eternal. The body is fulfilling its purpose as it dies, even if it is piece by piece.
4. The emotional/spiritual needs of a person last a lifetime; they do not end with illness or physical limitations.
5. Sacred worth is valued each time we allow the individual to express his true feelings and needs without fear of being criticized for feeling that way.

Sharing the gospel of hope and possibility with the aging is not always an easy task. The delight of doing so is how often the aging are out in front of the care giver, already finding ways to live out the challenge. Many of them have spent their lifetimes trying to heed the call, **'Come, follow me!'** There is arrogance in the assumption that because a person is old he is having difficulty doing so and needs "our" help. In some sense we all need the help of others to stay faithful, but to assume that is the case because of age is simply out of sync with the experience of too many care givers. How many of us marvel at the witness older adults make, growing old with grace and faithfulness. Sharing the gospel with the older adult is about witnessing to the person's continuing self-worth and value to God and to us. How we do that is of less importance than that we allow that insight to be a guiding principle in our ministry with this age group. So much around them denies this insight, largely because of social conditioning and blinders. It is the task of those who would speak for Jesus to see them as he sees them - whole and sacred!

How well I remember Mae. She was a member of the first congregation I served as a full-time associate pastor. After only a few weeks in that role, her family came to see me to ask a favor of me. Would I tell her that the time had come for her to move out of her home? The family had room and willingness for her to live with one of them. If she would not do so they were ready to help pay the expenses at a local "Home for Aging People" (a euphemism frequently used in those days). Too often it referred to a place where older adults felt isolated from the world and community they loved. They said, "We tried to tell her how much better it would be for her to move out of such a big house with so many stairs. "Suppose she falls one day and none of us know it? Suppose she gets sick without any of us knowing it? Legitimate concerns about a ninety plus year old woman! Or so a young pastor assumed! "Sure, I'll go sometime today."

Upon visiting Mae a lesson about assumptions was learned, especially assumptions about the ability of old people to be guided by their own spirituality. After hearing all the reasons why I agreed with her family, Mae pointed her finger at me and said true words.

"Young man you have a lot to learn if you are going to be a good pastor. You cannot just listen to my family. Listen to me! I am never alone in this house, God is always with me. If I fall, I fall. If I get sick, I get sick. If I die, I die. But I know I am never alone! You of all people should know that."

A chastened, but wiser, young man returned to the office that day. While the family surely had legitimate concerns, I surely would never make such assumptions again. Mae, if seemed to me, did not need help. Her family did! I did! We had missed the fact that Mae took her faith seriously and lived without fear. She felt whole and connected to her source of strength and therefore not alone. We needed to digest that and seek other ways to address the family's concerns. Mae was fine. Her own spiritual journey had seen to that,

Having told this story, let me be quick to add that in some sense we all need the help of others, but to assume that age alone requires intervention is simply out of sync with reality. Many older adults grow old 'alone' with grace and faithfulness. Sharing the gospel with older adults is about witnessing to their continuing self-worth and value to God and to us. How we do so is less important than that we allow that insight to be our guiding principle in ministry with this age group. So much around them denies this insight, largely because of social conditioning and blinders. It is the task of those who do such ministry to see them as God sees them – as whole and sacred.

For Further Thought

This section talks about offering a holistic gospel. How do you understand that phrase? What are the implications for those engaged in a ministry with older adults? Specifically, how might your understanding of this phrase change the way you see the relationship between the one offering ministry and the one receiving it?

Have you been called upon to preach or witness to older adults? Can you relate to the writer's comments about challenging them when doing so? Where are the areas in which preaching (or witnessing) challenging words would be helpful to the older person's spiritual journey? What are some of the barriers to doing so?

Have you been asked to pray for someone? How did you feel about that? Did you feel adequate to the task? What is the difference between praying 'for' and praying 'with' someone?

Joanne Seltzer's poem is quoted. The writer was struck by the phrase "every family is holy." What do these words mean to you? How might your understanding of them affect the way you look at your relationships with aging people?

Mae's story caused the author to question his assumptions. Have you ever felt the need to reexamine any of your assumptions? How have your assumptions affected the way you care for and about the older person(s) in your life?

REPECTING THE RIGHT TO MAKE CHOICES

"My kids are coming to see me, as are their families."

Knowing that they lived out of state and usually came several times a year at planned moments. I wondered why his two daughters and their families were coming at the same time.

"I asked them to come," he said, "so that I could tell them that I have entered hospice care, which I have arranged on my own. My wife knows, but the kids do not, I want to tell them myself."

About a year earlier he and his wife, who has early Alzheimer's, had entered the Wicke Health Center, at Wesley Village. Aware of her disease and aware of his progressing congestive heart failure and his cancer, he had made those arrangements so that she would be cared for in a familiar setting when he died. He was always honest about life and death, facing all the changes brought. He knew his treatment for the congestive heart failure and for the cancer was not working. Rather than put his family through the wrenching decision making about how to respond to that fact, he made his decision independently. His decision to enter hospice care did not come as a surprise.

What did come as a surprise were the people who suggested that he should not have been allowed to make that decision. They had different reasons, but the underlying theme was that at 94 years of age someone else should be making his decisions.

There was a presumption that older adults cannot and should not be making their own decisions. I see and experience this attitude quite frequently as I visit with family members and friends of residents in our community. Too many of them see their aging loved one as a child to be parented, rather than as a mature adult. They often confuse physical limitations with mental and spiritual limitations. Each and every time I feel this is the situation I am compelled to remind them that age is not a determining factor in making decisions. Competency, cognitive ability, mental and emotional health are the determining factors! He was perfectly able to make the decision he made. There was nothing wrong with him cognitively, emotionally or spiritually - despite his physical ailments and limitations. I applaud his courage and honesty.

In doing ministry with and for older adults, pastors and lay people have a great deal of influence with other people. We need to spread the word in this regard. We need to encourage family members and friends of older people not to limit them more than they need to be. We need to respect them as whole people, even if their bodies are failing them. To do less is to infantilize them and take an important piece of their self-worth from them - surely not a goal of ministry at any level.

While it may be easy to agree in principle that the goal of ministry with older adults begins with seeing them as whole and sacred, it is not always easy to do so in our caring for them. As they advance in years their ability to decide often becomes labored and never-ending. Their choices often seem wrong and unwise. At least to those who love them. Forgetfulness, for some, causes them to neglect their daily routines, most especially which pills to take. Living alone, as many of them do, many eat inadequately. Aches and pains sometimes keep them indoors and inactive. Many a loved one faces the dilemma of how to care for Mom or Dad when these times arrive. "How do I respect her rights as a human being I love and still see that her needs are met safely?" In one way or another this is the question of aging which is the most difficult to deal with for a care giver, be it a family member, a pastor, a caring lay minister, or any other concerned person. When the question arises it becomes too easy to return to "rational" ways of handling the situation, rather than "emotional" ways. It becomes too easy to do what is "best" for Dad, neglecting the emotional and spiritual needs that are also important. It is too easy to pretend the other side of the coin does not exist, the side which reveals the person within the "problem" at hand. The older adult, despite his situation does not stop having feelings, dreams, fears and such just because he is old. These need to be considered as well as safety and physical health issues!

Perhaps there is no more terrifying experience for an older adult than having to leave familiar surroundings, a house filled with memories, "artifacts" of a life, a street filled with friendly faces and the like. And perhaps there is no more terrifying experience for an adult child than having to leave that parent in current surroundings. Often the older adult fears the loss of control, and the "downsizing" of memories. They often cannot hear a loved one say anything that reminds them of what they already know: "I am entering the last phase of my life." The other literally fears for the safety and well being of a parent, now less capable physically and often mentally. It is a case of competing fears! The question is "how do we deal with the situation in a way that answers both fears?" There is likely no perfect answer or way around this dilemma. But experiences reveal that workable solutions are available. These solutions are dependent upon so many factors, all of them situational. No one answer is right for everyone.

How "unsafe" is the older adult in reality?" Are other caring adults (who are not emotionally attached to the person) seeing the same dangers and problems?

How limited is the person? What does the doctor say? Would an aide help?

Is living with an adult child better than an assisted living situation? Has the relationship between the two been such as to support the living arrangements?

Whose need is being met? Is it about the adult child's peace of mind more than about the care and comfort of the parent?

Tough questions! But without careful, prayer filled, attention to them many avoidable problems arise. Small groups exploring issues of aging, Biblical understandings about aging and family dynamics (preached and taught) help prepare young and old for facing aging. Supportive church ministries to/with older adults go a long way in helping the process, regardless the decision to move "Mom" or to leave her in her own home.

Caring for an older adult is a difficult task. But being an older adult is also a difficult task. How much better for everyone if we wrestle with the issues before they arise? Who better to lead us to clearer, practical applications of our faith in such matters than the church?

Our culture has not taught us how to deal with these difficult questions. Fortunately there are exceptions to this arising more and more frequently. As our society ages, moving for the first time to having more people over sixty-five than it has people under twenty-one is forcing these question to the forefront. Hospitals, nursing homes, assisted living facilities, long term care institutions, are now dealing with them as never before. Rising costs for such institutional settings, decreasing insurance benefits to pay these costs, an increasing life span, all drive these questions. There is growing emphasis on the questions "what is best for the aging person," and "what that older person wants in the way of care?" Two questions that at first blush seem to be at odds with each other, but which I believe are intertwined. For if the care plan is not what the older person wants, the question has to asked, is it really what is best? Not easy questions to answer, but in every situation they are questions that must be addressed.

One way to answer them is found in the ever growing "pre-planning" movement. Living Wills, Advanced Medical Directives and the like are facts of life, and well needed. But they are not enough for they tend to address the physical realities, but not the emotional and spiritual realities, that together make a whole person. Churches would do well to spend time and effort, using their foundation of faith as their basis, on these questions.

How many family members and others who care for older adults recognize this next situation? It speaks about insurance, but more so about the need to let others know what we find important to us before we are unable to do so.

"It was only after my mother died that we realized she had long term health insurance. It would have made things a lot easier if we had known beforehand. We never had to place her in a nursing home, but we sure worried about how we would pay for it if the need would have arisen."

This daughter's story is all too typical. Too often older adults (for a variety of reasons) do not share a clear list of information a caregiver would need to meet the needs of a sick or incompetent older adult. When crises come, family members, or friends, are often left without the information required to do the best that is possible for their loved one.

Increasingly it is not enough to have a living will, a medical proxy or someone with the power of attorney. Insurance information, both health and life, are important pieces of information for a caregiver. Wants and wishes about care, about location of health care facilities, doctor and hospital preferences are valuable tools for a caregiver.

What a vital ministry it would be if churches would offer occasional sessions of planning for crises of illness and disability! Creating a list with the older adult to be kept on file at the church, as well as sharing this list with the designated caregiver would offer comfort to all concerned.

In a time of high costs, increased options, and better informed older adults, and desire to have our wishes followed, it is necessary to plan ahead and to make a list that is as specific as possible.

What better setting to make these choices than within the community of faith, where our beliefs about life and death are considered important? What better setting than the church which sees beyond the temporal and envisions death as a gateway rather than a closed door?

Forging a ministry that looks at the issues surrounding aging before memory loss, cognitive disabilities and such set in allows the possibility that the older adult will be heard, even if she is no longer capable of doing so. By making a discussion of these issues a part of one's faith journey, a person can wrestle with the theological and spiritual concerns such issues raise. A person can make his beliefs about life, illness and death on the basis of his own faith, prayerfully and faithfully. He can do so while everyone concerned knows "he knows what he is doing." This can greatly ease the transition from one phase of life to the next, both for the individual and for the caregiver. What a relief it is for a family member to say, and to know the truth of the statement, "this is how Mom would want to be treated."

Even when we know what an older person wishes however, following those wishes does not mean she will not have to deal with loss and grief. The decision to make changes at any age is one of the most traumatic events in life. While it can, and often is, coupled with a sense of joy and anticipation, it is also tinged with loss and grief. This sense of loss and grief often drives the decision making process. Not recognizing this leads many a care giver to high levels of frustration and many an older person to higher levels of frustration born of feeling that "no one really understands what I am facing." This often leads to a stalemate, as the older adult digs in the heels and becomes unbending and the caregiver becomes frustrated and angry, leaving everyone with an inability to make the best decision possible. As decisions concerning long term care, either within one's own home or some other place, arise, forgetting the whole person again becomes problematic. The issue is not just what is safe for a person; it is also what will address all the concerns of a whole human being? Spiritual and emotional well being, as we have noted before, are as important as the physical well being of a person. Addressing only the physical leads to grief, anger, and frustration, because no matter how much we might want to pretend otherwise, change of any kind involves having to let go of the familiar and walking a new path. Older people's feelings about such things are often ignored, even though they are the ones who have to walk the new path. Adult children who recognize this and choose to walk it as a partner with the loved one finds both their own grief and frustration and their loved one's lessens as a result.

Many a transition goes badly because we do not recognize the grieving an older adult must face in order to make a change. We turn now to a discussion of the different losses faced by older adults, the toll grief takes on them, and some ways of working through it with them in a partnering way.

For Further Thought

It is often difficult for caregivers to acknowledge that the older adult, unless significantly cognitively impaired, has an inherent right to make her own decisions regarding care and treatment and of dealing with issues of aging. It often seems as if "we know better than Mom. Our only concern is what is in her best interest." Or so we tell ourselves? Does anyone have the right to make decisions for someone else just because they might make a different decision than we would?

Is it ever justifiable to make decisions that are against the wishes of the other person? What might be the criteria for doing so?

Is there a definable age at which a person should no longer make important decisions? If there is not an age per se are there definable events that might negate the right to make personal decisions? What might some of those events be?

The author mentions advanced directives, living wills and such as means of preserving the person's right to make choices. Are there ways churches and other caring institutions can enhance the possibility of people making sure their voices are always heard and their wishes followed?

Have you had a conversation about your long term wishes and followed through on making sure they are known and followed?

GRIEF AND LOSS

Enid Shomer, whose poem appears in **When I Am An Old Woman I shall Wear Purple** (Martz, op.cit), points poignantly to one of the more traumatic changes of all.

> *When I leave,*
> *the nurse is helping her change for the evening*
> *A small virtue to want to die*
> *as she lived: in a good*
> *silk dress, some detail*
> *like bugle beads*
> *at the collar and cuffs.*

Ministering to and with older adults constantly reminds me of perhaps the biggest loss so many of them face. It is the loss of the familiar routines of their lives. The ability to have breakfast when and if they want it! The choice to dress before breakfast or after! The routine of seeing neighbors and friends on a regular basis! The daily routine phone call to an adult child! So many bits and pieces - seemingly insignificant - that help define a life! So many important bits and pieces not always available to the older adult, made difficult by the need for help that can only be addressed in a nursing home, an assisted living facility, a move to an adult child's home, or a need to rely on aides who come at unfamiliar times.

"A small virtue to want to die as she lived..." Ministry to/with older adults requires us to be sensitive to this virtue. Older adults are not just being stubborn when they resist change. The routines of their lives are as important to them as ours are to us. Anything we can do to enable them to retain these routines is good ministry. Clergy and concerned lay people can advocate with family members to be sensitive to this need. Family members can be helped to see that Mom or Dad has a right to be an integral part of any change in their lives, to the fullest extent possible. What their "stubborn" parent or family member is asking is nothing other than we would ask in the same situation. "Do unto others as you would want others to do unto you" is once again a maxim to live by as we seek to relate and minister to the aging - be they family members, church members, or neighbors.

Preserving as many routines for the older adult as possible will make whatever changes are necessary easier to accept. It will enable the person to adapt more quickly to the new emerging routines and return more readily to living as fully as possible.

Keeping this sensitivity before us will make ministry to the whole person more likely to happen. Without it, we too easily fall into dealing with the physical needs and neglecting the emotional and spiritual needs. Empowering the aging to make their own decisions (as much as they are able), giving them a voice as to when and where they will relocate, allowing them to choose to bring with them as many familiar items as space will allow, allowing them to select bed spreads, pillows, etc. are all tools to use in assisting a change in relocation. All of them are attitudes of partnering rather than parenting. All of them suggest we empathize with the pain of making changes. All of them suggest we share the loss of the familiar with them.

There is no way to sugar coat the reality! Age brings changes, many of them unwanted and fearsome. Relocating is never easy. But it is made easier if the one making the move knows the love and support, the empathy and patience of a loved one. Being that person for someone else is a way of affirming the incarnation. It is a way of remembering that God was in Christ and, as those who follow Christ, helping to make God visible through us. We are the hands of God, and often the one way older adults experience the presence of God. If aging people do not experience that in those who care for them, the loneliness, the sadness, the grief will deepen. They will feel 'out of control' and be unlikely to receive the gospel promise of abundant life in their current situation.

In fact, if an aging person feels she is making the changes forced on her by circumstances beyond her control; if she feels that nothing will ever feel right again; and that no one really understands, she will likely exhibit some 'bad' behavior. One of these is often "crabbiness." How often family members have said "We just don't understand why Mom is so crabby, it is not how she used to be!" And how often I want to respond, "Don't you get it, she's so crabby because you don't understand!" But I usually just listen as they follow their thoughts, which often go something like this. "We've done everything we could to find a nice place for her, we sorted her belongings for her, we packed for her, we did everything we could to make the move easier. Why is she so crabby and unappreciative?"

"Crabby old people!" How often I encounter that expression! How often I encounter older people, some of whom are indeed "crabby." What I don't see often enough in my ministry with older adults is visitors and family members taking time to understand the "perceived" crabbiness. Because there is always an underlying reason for it and very often it is not the reason raised by the older adult.

Older adults have experienced cumulative losses in their lives. Spouses have died, adult children have moved away, living arrangements have been changed, and friends who once made up their support system have died or become ill. Often they can no longer attend church as they once did. They have to rely on others to do things they once did for themselves and others. The familiar rhythms are gone! As with people of every age when they do not face and deal with the losses of their lives, they get stuck in anger, often unnamed and unrecognized. I'm constantly amazed at how much grief goes unseen in the older adult. It is often masked with medicine and an easy dismissal such as "old people just get that way, I guess. I suppose when I'm old I'll be crabby too." Crabbiness can be a sign of unresolved grief and be a sign of someone stuck at the anger stage.

How a ministry of listening is needed with older people! Exploring the losses of their lives with them in a caring non-judgmental way helps the grieving process. When visiting a 'crabby' old person, encourage conversation about his life. When a loss is mentioned ask sensitive questions. "I can't imagine losing a spouse after so many years together. I wonder how you got through it?" "You lived in that house for fifty-five years. I've never lived anywhere that long. What was it like to leave it?" Ask questions that reveal empathy, not easy answers. Listen to the responses! You're now doing ministry of listening and it is a healing ministry.

When doing ministry with older adults it is important be sensitive to their moods. They tell us something about the physical and spiritual health of the person. Pay attention to the crabbiness, it may be a sign of grief that might be helped by empathetic listening. Take the example of Jesus with you, the example of one who was slow to judge, but quick to pay attention to the person.

Dealing with loss and change can be eased! It cannot and should not be avoided. It does not have to be the fearful thing it usually is! No matter how traumatic or painful dealing with loss and change may be, a whole and healthy person depends on doing so! Those caring for and those ministering to an older adult do him no favor by avoiding the subject. They simply decrease the likelihood of moving on to a renewed sense of wholeness. However it cannot be forced! It must come naturally, born out of a relationship of trust. That kind of relationship is built by exhibiting empathetic, listening behavior, behavior that is responsive to the needs of a whole person. One of the better examples of this type of behavior is being modeled where I do ministry.

We are engaged in a major renovation of our resident apartments at the United Methodist Homes. Needless to say it is a difficult process for the residents who need to be moved to another apartment while their apartment is gutted and rebuilt. The other day our administrator remarked that he had greatly underestimated the ability of our residents to adjust to these necessary moves. He was rightly concerned that moving people in their eighties and nineties - even temporarily - would be more traumatic than some would tolerate. But the residents seem to be coping well.

What happened, we wondered? Why is this aged population dealing so well with forced change, with the inevitable noise and dirt that accompanies such projects, and with the unknowable date of when they can move back to their "own" apartments? Indeed why are some of them even enjoying their new surroundings?

We think we know! First of all, before each move, we took pictures of each apartment showing the details of where pictures were hung, clothing was stored, and furniture was placed. To the best of our ability the temporary apartments were arranged accordingly. The residents know that when they move back to their own place it will be arranged the same way again, if that is what they want. Second we constantly acknowledge how difficult the change must be and commend them on how well they are coping. And third, as a staff, we have made ourselves available to anyone at anytime who is having a concern with the process.

It strikes me, that as people age and life forces changes on them, these are things to remember. Change at best is difficult for some and at worst very traumatic for others. Familiar things arranged in a familiar pattern helps many a transition. Acknowledging how difficult it is allows the person to know that their feelings of displacement and loss are normal. Commending a person on her adjustment goes a long way in encouraging the process. It is a way of saying, 'I know you can do it. You have what it takes!" Being available through a time of change relieves the loneliness and sense of 'no one cares what I'm going through.'

Pastors, concerned lay people and family do well to remember the ministry of caring is about meeting people where they are and providing the encouragement and wherewithal to move on. It is too easy to simply expect the older adult to 'be realistic,' and to face the truth. It is too easy to say, 'You're intelligent, you know you must make this *change.' A caring ministry helps to create an environment in which change - even if not welcomed - is seen as acceptable and workable.*

Give your older loved ones the gift of understanding the difficulty of facing unwanted changes in their lives and the gift of your presence and support. Most will find what they need in that and begin to adjust.

Once again the impetus for that is more than simple human sympathy and kindness, as important as that is. The goal of ministry with older adults is wholeness. That cannot be found if a person does not see possibility before him, however limited that possibility may be! Without possibility - Christians know it better by its other name, hope - there is no incentive to adjust. Why not just sit back and wait for the inevitable, becomes the question for someone without hope? If we are serious about challenging the aging to claim the whole gospel, including the possibility of life beyond death, we will create environments which offer a taste of that life beyond death in the here and now. A person who experiences newness of life at any age experiences a taste of resurrected living. Being with a person, creating an environment of possibilities enhances the chances of that new life occurring. Grief and loss give way to hope when a person knows he has choices, knows he can still contribute to the larger community, when he senses that his life's circumstances may be changing, but that his value has not been diminished.

A glimpse of this process taking place became clear very recently. In our assisted living facility we have a painting class, as we do in our other facilities as well. Mary was showing me the oil paintings she had recently done. I was stunned! They were quite good! What stunned me was that Mary had even attended the class. When I first met her she appeared resigned to be in an assisted living community, but not happy about it. It was not, she had said, her first choice. She had come reluctantly because she could not see any other way of managing her life. Her medical issues were uppermost in her mind. She talked about them constantly. Even though encouraged to become involved in that community she had resisted. "What made you go to the class?" "I was bored and going crazy so I figured I'd give it a try. Was I surprised to discover I had talent! Had I not been here I might never have known. Who would have thought a woman over eighty would discover a new talent and a new love?'

Who? The one in whose name we do ministry, the one who called people of every age to abundant living! That is who! Ministering to older adults is about calling them to live out this call, to accept this offer. How we do that is as varied as the person with whom we are dealing, but our task is to create environments and relationships in which the aging might discover "a new talent and a new love." It is not easy, it does not always happen, but it becomes more likely when we keep the goal in mind, when we challenge the aging to see possibility and hope in every circumstance of their lives.

A glimpse into how this challenge might be posed follows!

"It is not the race she chose but, by God, it is the race she was in, so she ran it as well as she could." Nancy Grace, a United Methodist and lawyer of television fame, used this line as a theme of a keynote address to the United Methodist Association at a recent Conference in Cambridge, MA. She told the story of a friend who entered a race to be run in Central Park in NYC. So anxious was she to run the race for the first time, and just recovering from a serious illness, she arrived quite early. A few hours, in fact! Sometime after arriving people started lining up for a race. Thinking it was the one she planned to run, she lined up as well. Hearing the starting gun, she began running. Soon she noticed the signs along the way - one mile, two mile, three mile. She began thinking 'this is a longer race than I planned on running.' But she did not stop! She pushed on, eventually finishing the race, having run further than she had ever done before. At which time she discovered what she already suspected; she had entered the 'wrong race.' The one she had prepared for was scheduled for a much later start than the one she actually ran.

Nancy Grace's point was that people in health and other caring ministries often find they are "running a race for which they did not sign up." I could not help relating this insight to many older adults who I know and have come to love. Many of them would understand her observation. Life often leads down unexpected paths, often leads to a longer, more difficult race than they might have thought or chosen.

The task, the challenge of ministry, with such people is to challenge, to inspire, to witness to this most faithful insight. Ultimately we do not choose the circumstances of our lives, they choose us. The task is to help them see Paul's vision:

> *"Nothing in all creation can separate us from the love of God in Christ Jesus our Lord"*
>
> *"I can do all things through him who strengthens me".*

The task of such ministry is to witness that it is not the circumstances that determine the meaning of our lives, it is the response to those circumstances that do. It is about encouraging possibility, even while acknowledging limitations. It is not about platitudes. "Everything will be okay, just wait and see." It is not about raising false expectations. It is about calling the older adults with whom we minister to declare: "It is not the race I chose but, by God, it is the race I am in. I will run it as well as I can."

How we do that happens in a variety of ways. Our theology, our personalities, our abilities, will lead us to ways that fit us. The extent to which we do so determines the effectiveness of our ministry with older adults. Regardless their limitations they have much to offer their churches, their communities, their families, their institutional settings, their roommates, etc. Not to challenge them to do so is to tell them that they no longer are valued persons in our midst. So struggle with ways to witness and inspire the older adults in your midst. The meaning of their remaining days may depend on it.

Grief and loss do give way to hope and possibility when supportive environments and relationships are in place. Hope and possibility lead to the abundant life which the gospel offers to all. A ministry of healing, a ministry to the whole person, which honestly addresses grief and loss through listening to the pain that accompanies them, is a holistic ministry, one worthy of the calling to **"Come, follow me!"** It is a ministry which encourages the aging **"to run the course with faith."**

There are a variety of ways to do this! Is our ministry with/for groups of older adults? Is it with individuals? Are these older adults physically and cognitively in good health? Is the individual in good health? What are the interests, the needs, the joys, the sorrows of those with/for whom we are ministering? What can they still do to be of service to the larger community - pray, phone a lonely person, write notes, be hospitable to the stranger in their midst? Challenging them to claim abundant life has to allow ways for serving others. Is that not the lesson Jesus taught so well and so often? No one size or approach to ministry will fit. There is no short cut to caring for a whole person or group if we don't know them as such. There is no end run around the need to build care-filled, honest, listening, partnering relationships. This ministry is not all about serious work. It is not just about meeting needs, spiritual or physical. It is about affirming the gift of aging as something to be claimed and welcomed. With age comes a freedom unknown in younger years. The stress of building careers, families, homes and other concerns are no longer there. Having found ways to cope with these stress factors they have developed ways to deal with the issues of later years. A task of those caring for/about them is to help them see they have this ability, already demonstrated by the fact they have attained advanced years. Knowing that gives them a freedom to pursue other interests. What is often missing is the awareness that despite the limitations which often come with age, there is this freedom to rediscover the self that has, at times, been buried under the pressures of everyday living.

It is to this freedom, this time of new possibility that we now turn. The problem is that we often miss this freedom because of our need to concentrate on the issues of aging. We often miss it because even the ones to whom and with whom we minister do not want to acknowledge the fact of aging. So conditioned are we to seeing age through our culture's prism that we pretend it is not happening until circumstances force us to do so. Typical of this way of seeing was a conversation I had recently.

I remarked "I guess we're both just getting old." The immediate response was "Don't say that word!" It is an all too typical response or feeling. In a time when youth sells, where Botox, anti-wrinkle creams, and plastic surgery are big business the word 'old' has a negative connotation. How often do we hear dismissively, "he's just old?" We seem to have lost a sense of wonder and respect for the aging process.

Our faith affirms "So we do not lose heart. Though our outer nature is wasting away, our inner nature is being renewed every day." (2Corinthians 4:16) Christian ministry to and with older adults is about addressing this reality. It sees the physical and cognitive changes that come with aging. It sees the limitations age brings. And it rightly addresses the physical and cognitive changes in practical ways. This is the area in which decisions related to housing, physical care, and medical attention is addressed. But Christian ministry does not stop there. It seeks ways to explore how the inner nature is being renewed, ways in which it can work with the Holy Spirit in tapping into the continuing value of the aging person.

Christian ministry is not afraid to say the word "old." In fact, it says it with respect. The older person of faith has lived and experienced so many renewals in her life. She has much to teach the rest of the community about living in grace, about reliance on God's love. The older person of faith, despite the other areas of aging, is a necessary and valuable member of any community. Christian ministry keeps this truth in front of the aging individual and the community at large.

If we cannot keep this insight before us, our older adult ministry is doomed to fail in its goal to affirm a whole person. If we forget this insight, we will never reach the point of celebrating the gift of aging. Even writing these last four words gives me pause. **The gift of aging!** I am too aware of the other side of the coin, too aware of how often age brings diminished abilities on so many levels. I am too aware of how often the following conversation has taken place.

"Jim, Mom is just waiting to die. There is nothing wrong with her other than the usual complaints of old age. But she won't do anything. She just sits in her room, day after day. She won't come to family functions. She won't participate in the activities at the assisted facility where she lives. I'm at my wit's end. I don't know how to motivate her to do something."

A very common concern of those who care for an aging loved one! As is the response I hear so often from the older adult caught in this behavior pattern. "What's the use of getting involved? I'm going to die soon and so is everyone else around me. I've lived my life. Now all that is left is memories and waiting."

We need to work to reclaim aging as a time of beauty and possibility, a time for new insights and directions. It is not an easy task! It is difficult to see that aging can be a period of remarkable growth and abundant living. It is difficult to claim the freedom from so many stresses and concerns of the younger years, when we are conditioned to see only the problems of aging. In fact it is even more difficult when we misread what the aging are saying to us.

"She used to be so active. All she does now is sit. She doesn't even knit or crochet any more. She won't read. She doesn't want company and she used to love having visitors. It makes me so angry and frustrated. There is no reason for her to behave this way. What do I do about that? I am at my wits end. I've tried everything to help her adjust to her new surroundings."

Unfortunately these are familiar words, uttered frequently by frustrated family members who say, "I just don't understand my Mom. She just isn't who she used to be."

The problem is that she is quite likely exactly who she has always been, with one big exception. Moving to a new location, separated from familiar settings, surrounded by strangers, missing her old homestead, may have been one loss too many. So it seems to many an older adult who finds herself in this situation. That sense of feeling one loss too many is not an uncommon experience as we age, even if we remain where we feel most comfortable. It is not the moving in and of itself that is the problem. It is the number of losses and the frequency with which they seem to come as we age that is the issue. Seeing Mom as intractable is more often than not the problem. A lack of understanding the dynamics is!

Coupled with this sense of loss can be a depression, which is often not recognized. That can lead to an unwillingness of an older adult to stay engaged, which can lead to a sense of isolation, which in turn can lead to boredom and dissatisfaction. If these issues are not addressed they are likely to worsen. A skilled professional, trained in dealing with the issues of older people is often very useful. Most older adults adjust to changes in due time, if they are in a supportive environment and have a caring support system as they find their way to new life. There is a way to know the difference between a 'normal' missing their old way of life and clinical depression. Using a professional is always wise if there is any doubt. It is not an easy thing to deal with, nor is the path for doing so always clear. But there are tactics that are helpful once we are sure we are not dealing with clinical issues.

A common result of grief and loss is often an ensuing sense of loss and boredom. By no means do all older adults have these feelings. It is amazing, despite their mounting losses, older adults usually handle changes creatively, bypassing much of the depression and loneliness and boredom. Some come to new settings and seem to adjust as they arrive. What's their secret? They are no different than the others, yet they quickly seem happy. How can this be? There are many reasons. Many have developed skills for coping with change over a lifetime. Many have not. But for those engaged in caring for those who are coping with change, there are some ways in which to create an environment in which change can more readily be embraced. One of these ways became clearer as I was driving grandchildren somewhere. There words, quite familiar to a father of six children, prompted a reflection of such matters.

"Are we there yet?" "I'm bored, there is nothing to do. Have you ever heard these words from a child? If you have raised children and have ever taken them for a ride, I guarantee you have heard them. When our children had all grown up, we thought we had heard them for the last time. But then along came the grandchildren! It tickled me to hear my daughter, who has three children of her own say, "I don't understand. They have their electronic games, movies and what have you – all of them in the car. Why do they get so restless?"

It's an age old question that probably dates back to similar conver-sations in the Stone Age, as our forbears traveled, looking for food and shelter. There is a restlessness about us that is real. We always seem to want that which we cannot have. We want things to be the way they 'used to be.' We want to be as physically able as we were. We want to live where we have always lived. No one wants to be confined in any way. Yet what do we do about the fact that we cannot always have these things?

Older adults are victims of this syndrome too. So much of their familiar routine is different. Abilities can change. Health can change. On the list goes! Often feeling sorry for themselves, they give way to idleness rather than finding a new way to be creative and alive. How do we enable those caught in this mood to deal with the inevitable changes that cause them to feel confined and limited? Whining and complaining doesn't help. Nor does listening patiently to them do so. Listening is important, but it is equally important to enable a different direction. Anyone who has ever spent time in a car with a youngster knows the art of doing just that.

"Let's play a new game! Let's see who can count the most red cars on the road!"

"Let's see who can go the longest without saying a word!"

My favorite antidote to the adult version of "I'm bored" is a method I use constantly in my ministry. Knowing that helping someone else always lifts one's Spirit, my antidote is to ask a question. "We really need someone to.... Would you do this for me? I keep a mental list of possibilities for volunteering at all times, offering the bored older adult a task he would be able to do. Simple acts, such as making an unexpected phone call or knocking on some lonely resident's door are among the requests. Getting a yes not only lifts the person's Spirit, it actually helps those around, creating an attitude of caring and sharing.

We need to find ways to proclaim aging as a time of new life tied less to the physical and more to the spiritual! Effective ministry to and with older adults begins with knowing that age is not a barrier to being relational and engaging with the world around us. It begins with seeing the older adult as having intrinsic value regardless her abilities or inabilities. Bessie was a perfect example of moving beyond boredom and loneliness. She had been through a rough couple of years. Within a short time she had been widowed and her siblings and her daughter had died. On top of that, she had moved from her own home into one of our assisted living communities. Her life had changed! Not an uncommon story! What is uncommon is that Bessie was usually smiling and engaged in activities, often in a service mode. Bessie loved to do for others.

She said once as she crocheted for our prayer shawl ministry, "I love to do this. It makes me feel good to be able to help someone else. It keeps me from dwelling on my own problems. I think about them while I'd crocheting, calling Bingo or whatever else. But they don't seem so overwhelming when I'm doing something for someone else.

Bessie was over 90 and spoke volumes about the importance of enabling possibilities for people as they age to serve. We often do not challenge them to remember we are called to serve. Age may change the ways in which we can do so, but it does not eliminate the importance of doing so. We make a mistake when we cater to their every need, especially if they are capable of meeting some of their needs by themselves. When we do cater too much, we create a sense of entitlement that denies their capabilities and leads to low self-esteem at best, and angry, demanding people at worst.

Effectively ministering with and to this group begins when they are challenged to do and to be the best they can, when we challenge them to give their time and talent in service to others. Doing so does not erase the losses of age. As Bessie knew all too well, the losses are real. Some are physical, some are emotional, and some are spiritual. All of these must be affirmed as part of the reality. Bessie also knew that serving others through volunteering created a better perspective and life.

The bottom line, despite any efforts a caregiver might make, only the individual can change the situation. The most anyone can do is to listen and empathetically acknowledge the validity of the feelings and suggest other scenarios. Older adults need to be challenged to see the continuing possibilities of service.

It is the single best way (that I know of) to deal with the issue of loneliness and boredom.

For Further Thought

Have you ever had to relocate and leave family, friends, familiar surroundings and routines? Can you identify the feelings of loss and grief you might have experienced even if you knew the move was for a good reason?

How do you suppose an older person, pushed to make a move by circumstance beyond his control, might feel? How would you cope in such a situation?

It is easy to forget that people's feelings and behaviors have roots somewhere. The writer suggests that 'crabby old people" may be suffering from unresolved grief over their losses. Have you ever experienced someone misreading your mood, someone not understanding your behavior or attitude? Have you ever wondered why "they just don't understand what I'm going through?" How might being in touch with that experience enable you to better respond to an older person exhibiting behaviors that seem inappropriate to you?

The story that Nancy Grace tells so provocatively opens doors to new understanding. All people have times when life calls them to go where they don't wish to go, or to do what they don't wish to do. Older people have such an experience frequently. How do you suppose they might feel in such circumstances?

Are there strategies for encouraging the aging to run an unwanted race with grace? What might they be?

Have you ever found yourself in a lonely period? Even when friends and family tried to see you through that period, did you find yourself rejecting their offers, preferring to 'work it through' on your own? Can you relate to older adults possibly having the same preference? If so, how might that affect the way you minister to and care for a lonely older adult?

CELEBRATING THE GIFT OF AGING

Each time I moved to a new church, I would spend the first few weeks attending the meeting of every group in the church. I went to the choir, the bell ringers, youth meetings, United Methodist Women groups (including all the circles), etc. One of the delightful surprises was my weekly visit to the sewing circle of a particular church. This was a group of women who met weekly to sew, knit, crochet, or just visit with one another, and of course, to have a rather sumptuous lunch. The youngest woman in the group was well into her seventies. Most were in their eighties and a few were in the nineties. I went with some trepidation. How would I survive a group of 'old ladies' who had been meeting together for almost sixty years? What would I say? What would I do? Would they find my presence intrusive? Despite the questions, I went anyway. Was I surprised! I enjoyed myself so much that I went to every sewing circle meeting that I could the whole time that I was the pastor.

What happened? For a while I didn't know what attracted me. But it eventually became apparent. These women had a deep concern for each other. They would phone each other daily to make sure all were well. They gave their "dues" to mission. They took food every week to someone they thought needed it. But more importantly, these women laughed a lot. Someone would mention an ache or a pain and soon someone would counter with a greater ache or pain and soon they would all be laughing at the "silliness" (as one woman called it) of old age. Intuitively they knew life is about community, about relationships, and not about aches and pains. They celebrated life! In the midst of infirmities they had discovered a deeper truth. They had discovered that joy and laughter and celebration were more powerful than any ache or pain. They celebrated life and they celebrated the God who sustained them. That group has remained, for me, a model of what the church should and could be. That group helped me understand the observation of Henri Nouwen.

"Is it possible for the elderly to find the wisdom of the child in a second playfulness? To care for the elderly means to play with the elderly in the hope that by playing together we will remind each other that dancing is more human than rushing, singing more human than shouting orders, poetry more human than 'The Wall Street Journal,' and prayers more human than tactful conversations. To play with the elderly is to recapture the truth that our sense of self is more important than what we achieve. It is not a regression to a childish state, but a progression to a second innocence in which the acquired skills and insights of adulthood are fully integrated. This second innocence can lead us to the mature and critical realization that celebration is the most human response to life."

Do we maybe spend too much time in our ministry with older adults dealing with 'their' issues and not enough time laughing and playing? Would we do better as churches to search for ways to celebrate God's gift of life at every age and stage? Is Nouwen leading us to find a new model for older adult ministries?

I am convinced that he is! There is much to celebrate, much to play and dance over as we age. But again, largely because we have allowed ourselves to believe that growing old is all about a failing body and mind, we pay too little attention to the spirit, the one aspect of our being that does not have to succumb to age. From our faith perspective it is this spirit that must respond to the call to **"Come, follow me."** If we continue to allow ourselves to see less than a whole person in the aging, we will miss a golden opportunity to encourage the Spirit to lead us into abundant life even as we age. Only our spirits can respond to the Spirit. Our spirits, much as our bodies and minds, respond much more willingly and positively if they are relaxed, peaceful and joyful. Ministry that provides opportunities for our spirits to relax, and experience peace and joy is ministry through which the Spirit can be heard and followed. Recreational activities are an important way of providing that opportunity. But what are 'good' recreational activities? As I said in the opening pages, not everyone enjoys Bingo or whatever the activity is. Finding activities that bring relaxation, peace and joy is not always an easy thing to do. The more we minister to the whole person, the more we know how unique individuals are - even about how to relax, what is enjoyable, what is renewing.

A growing awareness on the part of the activities departments where I work is a broader definition of recreation. Recreation for seniors has for a long time been about keeping them busy so they don't get bored. A worthy goal in itself! But it is not enough if we are going to address a whole person - body, mind, and spirit! We do well to remember the original meaning of the word, which is: to create a new thing from something old, to Re-create. It is a divinely inspired concept. The work of God according to our scriptures and tradition begins with an act of creating. As we read through those scriptures, as we parse the stories within the stories, we see God constantly allowing opportunities for the people to be re-created. Indeed the work of Jesus was largely about re-creating those who listened, those who followed him. It was the work of calling them to see and become all that they could, of calling them to claim anew the word of the creating God. Ministry which sees a whole person knows that simply keeping busy is not enough. In fact it may be blocking the joy of seeing new beginnings in every ending. Practically this may be played out in so many ways in churches, in institutional settings, and in our homes. Each person is unique and has a need to be challenged to serve according to specific ability, gift, interest or time. Some examples stand out! The danger with sharing them is that they be seen as "the way to provide re-creation for seniors." As we have noted several times there is always more than one way. One of the joys of working with older adults is that they will lead us in this area if we take the time to listen to them and to know them. For when we do, we learn the things where they have a passion, we learn their gifts and talents and we offer opportunities for these to be used for their re-creation.

Marie used to knit and crochet when she was active in her church, but with advancing age and some arthritis, she gradually had given up doing so. Eventually she had to enter the nursing home. She was invited to attend a weekly knitting group sponsored by the Director of Volunteer Services. She did not want to go because: "I don't remember how to knit, I'm slow and I make mistakes. Besides, who would I knit for, who would want something I made?" With some encouragement from staff, Marie started attending the group, learning how to knit again, and is now enjoying the socialization that goes with it. I see her nearly every afternoon. If she is not involved in some other activity, she is knitting. By her own admission, she is slow and still making mistakes. But she says, with a smile, "I have to get these scarves finished before next Christmas (eight months away as I write this). My grandchildren tell me my great grandchildren will love them." Seemingly a small thing! But it is large! Marie has a purpose for knitting. It is serving someone else, which gives her life added meaning and joy. And more importantly, because of her age, she has the gift of free time, time to use her talent and her interest.

Ministry with older adults is more effective when it faces this reality of aging. For most it brings free time, too much so for those who see no purpose in the free time. For most it brings physical limitations of one kind or another, often seen as reasons to stop living. Marie reminds us that when we make these things positive, rather than negative, we enable a vision of possibility and hope. That is something to celebrate!

I conduct worship and offer Holy Communion in all of our buildings. Recently the activity director in one of them called and asked if I would mind beginning the Service in her building a half hour earlier. She needed to be sure the room where we hold Worship Services would be empty early enough to allow for setting it up for a special dinner. The dinner would be attended by eight residents and ten sixth grade students and their teacher. The occasion was a joint discussion of a specific book the residents and students had read independently. The book, appropriate for sixth graders, was about the struggles of growing up. Ginny, the activities director, had enlisted residents who loved to read, but who often were alone in their reading, to share the reading project with the sixth graders. This involved reading the book and discussing it as a group before meeting with the youngsters, sharing their own struggles growing up (and growing old). When the day came for meeting together around the table, sharing a meal and experiences, one of the residents said, "I hope you don't mind being bumped to a different time slot, but it is important we meet with the kids. This is the only time they can come." She was excited and obviously aware of her value at that moment. She had something to share with the kids.

As I was leaving the building and the room was being reassembled for the dinner discussion, I met the sixth graders, along with their teacher, walking into the parking lot. They were vibrant, noisy, and excited. I stopped to thank them for coming and told them how much the residents were anxious to meet them. One of them said "I'm scared. I don't know any old people. I hope I say the right thing?" "Just be yourself," I suggested, they'll love your spirit."

The project called and challenged the older adults to abundant living, to be all they could be, if only for a short time. That is the goal! That moment of recreation did join in the divine work of creation. It surely made eight seniors more alive and animated and useful! And it surely made sixth graders more aware of the possibilities of growing old. Re-creation at its best!

One of the joys of aging is the ability to rediscover the joys known, all too often, only to the young. Interaction between generations is good for both the young and the old. It visually and experientially says everyone has something of value to share with someone else. The gift of vitality comes so naturally to the young. The gift of experience is only available as we age. How good it would be if we celebrated both young and old more often interactively as means of recreation! Churches, schools, nursing homes, assisted living facilities and such could all benefit from planning such activities.

When my daughter was seventeen I heard her tell her friends she was eighteen. When they left I said, 'Why did you tell them that, you are only seventeen?" "No Dad, I'm eighteen, I'll show you my driver's license." She proceeded to do so! Teenagers often have fake identification making them older than they really are?

Our children play dress-up, pretending to be older than they are. They play act the roles of important adults in their lives. They tell their parents: 'you're treating me like a baby,' hoping they'll treat them as adults before they really are. At four years of age, my granddaughter used to talk about 'when I'm five, I'm gonna....'

It takes a long time to become comfortable with who we are, a long time to become peaceful within, to accept on faith that life and all its ups and downs can be trusted to God. Jesus' admonition to become as children called his followers to this kind of youthfulness. Yet, we spend a large part of our childhood wanting to be older.

Only when we enter the older category do we begin to look back to younger days with longing. But we do so with a proviso! "If only I knew then what I know now." The older adult carries- a sense of history within, history that might have made things turn out differently if 'I knew then what I know now." An older adult cannot literally return to childhood or younger years, no one can! She can however look back and see the past from a new perspective. In many retirement homes, assisted living centers, nursing homes and such there are life review programs. Through life story telling, journaling and such, older adults are encouraged to review their lives. They are encouraged to discover that their story is incomplete. They begin to see they still have a present and a future and that they have learned valuable lessons along the way, most especially that life can (must) be trusted to God. These lessons will help them deal with the present as it unfolds. It is a fascinating endeavor in which the United Methodist Homes is actively participating.

I see lives changed as hope is renewed and the older adult grabs hold of the reality that life is not over. How often I am asked to visit our churches to talk about older adult ministries and find myself wishing they would pay more attention to life review. Rather than bemoaning the older adult's tendency to dwell in the past, how much more productive it would be to encourage revisiting the past, relearning its lessons and applying them in the present. Even though they are unaware of the fact, older adults have learned to move on, have learned they have the resources to cope with life's changes. They have learned lessons people of every age would do well to learn. They are a valuable resource and we would serve them and ourselves better if we found ways to let them share their life's lessons.

There is clearly a ministry from older adults that the Church and community have often missed because of the focus on doing ministry for them. This age group has experienced life in all it dimensions - its joys and its sorrows, its successes and its perceived failures, its hope and its despair. In that experience they have largely found ways to cope and to grow. They have much to teach the rest of us about living and moving on through all the phases of life. We miss much of what they have to teach us because of entrenched attitudes about aging. We too often allow ourselves to miss the unique gift this group offers to us. I remember so well the woman who, in her nineties, terminally ill with cancer, accepted the proposal from another ninety something year old to be married. Her friends and family thought she was out of her mind for doing so. Why would anyone in her situation even consider doing so? Why? I asked her that question and was forced to grow by her answer. "Because," she said, "life is for living, not for waiting to die. I know I don't have a long time to live, but there is no reason to stop doing so until God says it is time." I could not disagree with her reasoning or her theology. Her attitude was one of hope filled living, one that accepted the reality of finite time, but which also embraced life as a gift to be lived abundantly. She reminded me that ministry to and with older adults is about seeing life holistically, seeing life as filled with ever expanding possibility. Not to remember that is to be unable to see the older adult as a whole person, rather than a frail, ill, disabled member of the human family.

Ministry to and with older adults is about affirming the message that life is to be lived abundantly. It is to celebrate the possibilities so often lost in our vision of the aging. Ministry with the aging is not always serious business. It is often cause for joy and laughter as we marvel at the "silliness" of old age that limits its vision to diminishment rather than expanding possibilities. It is cause for joy as we embrace the message of the gospel that God has a place and a role for everyone, regardless of age or disability. Celebration of life as a gift in whatever form it comes is the bottom line of such ministry. We lose sight of that fact at the cost of effectiveness in our ministry with the aging. A reminder of what the power of that call came from my mother's doctor who one day listened to her complaints (which she usually did not offer) about her various aches and pains. He said, *"There is nothing wrong. Marion, you're just old!"*

I chuckle even writing these words, remembering her response to the Doctor's statement. As she came out of his office she was chuckling, which was followed by full-fledged laughter. "How could I have missed it? He said I was just old. There is nothing wrong with me." It was a relief to her. Her feelings were normal. They were part of the aging process. She was content with that. That episode led to the following thoughts.

Getting older often brings aches and pains in places we don't even know we have. They obviously need to be diagnosed by a doctor before simply dismissing them. But there is relief in knowing, "Marion, you're just old." There is honesty and realism. There is relief in knowing that aging is normal and as such no reason to sit and fret, obsessing over what we cannot change.

The doctor redirected my mother. He led her back to her normal attitude of enjoying every moment of her life. Even when the aches and pains would become more pronounced she did not worry. She would, at such moments, often smile and remark, "I guess he was right. I am just old."

What a departure from so many peoples' approach to aging! How often someone says, "Don't say that word to me. I don't want to be old. How often I say, "Why not? Being old is not a disease to be avoided! We all get there someday if we live long enough." Pastor, family members and other caregivers do a person a disservice by not acknowledging the reality. Being old is not a curse. It is simply a new phase of life. It can be full and meaningful if we do not run from it or skirt the issues it brings, if we see it as off limits for discussion. The truth is that aging often brings limitations we did not have before, but that does not mean it is not rife with possibilities for new experiences and new possibilities for growth. These will not be explored and discovered without first acknowledging, "Marion, you're just old."

Emphasizing only the negative aspects of age is too pervasive. It is time those involved in caring for and about the aging embrace the fact of 'getting old and begin celebrating and witnessing to its possibilities.

For Further Thought

So much of our culture is youth or young oriented. It is easy to fall into believing that old age is something to be avoided or postponed for as long as possible. There is a lot of ignoring the possibilities of aging. Have you ever considered that getting old is a cause to celebrate – not celebrating in the sense that someone you love has had his 90th birthday – but in the sense that you are heading toward old age as well? What are your inner most feelings about that reality? Do you have any fears about it? Do you anticipate with hopefulness and joy? How might acknowledging these feelings help you relate to the older person in your life?

The story is told about the older person in the author's congregation who laughed at "the silliness of old age." What thoughts did you have when first hearing that expression? Is there 'silliness' to old age? Is that a good thing or a bad thing?

"Marion, you're just old." Did you respond in any way to this diagnosis of the author's mother? What were your feelings? Was the doctor on to something important is saying what he did? How does his statement challenge our culture's general attitude regarding old age? How does it challenge your vision of old age?

USING HUMOR IN MINISTRY WITH OLDER ADULTS

Betty was in her early eighties, recently widowed and terminally ill with cancer. For reasons known only to her, she loved me and allowed me to know her as few others did. Most people saw her as a 'loner.' When it came time for her to enter a nursing home, I went with her and spent quite some time as she settled in. As I was getting ready to leave she began sobbing and asked if I would stay the night with her. Knowing she appreciated my sense of humor and knowing she loved my wife as much as she loved me, I said to her: "Let me get this right. You are asking me to spend the night with you. You're sick! You're over eighty years old and will fall asleep as soon as the lights go out. And you're asking me to stay knowing I can go home to my beautiful wife, who loves me as much as you do and who will not fall asleep as soon as the lights go out. Betty, what choice do I have? I have to go home." Midst a widening grin, she said, "You always did know how to make a girl feel good. Go home to your wife and come see me tomorrow."

Humor had defused a tough situation and had alleviated some fear, as well as allowed the truth to be spoken. Betty had to stay in that nursing home and I had to go home. The next day Betty was still *chuckling when she said, "Darn you, I fell asleep last night laughing at what you said. I even feel better this morning."*

There is something about laughter and humor that releases stress and opens up new possibilities. Humor changes our perspective. Try being angry while you are laughing! Try being mean spirited while someone is tickling your funny bone! It cannot be done. If we want to create a healing environment, laughter needs to be a common occurrence. Humor opens the door to finding joy in adversity (which I believe is a most appropriate use of humor.)

Don't be afraid to use humor when ministering with/to older adults. However, follow a few guidelines in doing so!

1. *Be sensitive to the situation.*
2. *Be sensitive to the person(s) involved. (I knew Betty would enjoy my response.)*
3. *If you wonder if a particular use of humor will be received badly, don't use it. It is likely inappropriate.*
4. *Never use humor out of context! A joke is often misunderstood. Humor should respond to the situation at hand.*
5. *Never use humor as a put down or as a way to deny feelings (yours or the person you are with.)*
6. *Use humor only if it will serve its purpose, relieving stress and opening new possibilities.*

Because older adults are a product of our culture they often approach their aging with a sense of dread and seriousness. Concerns about health, insurance and disabilities often become the reference points for them. There is little room for seeing the 'silliness' of aging with such reference points. Humor serves a useful purpose when carefully used. The old adage that laughter is good medicine applies to the aging as well as it does to any other age group. There is too much gloom and doom in conversations with the older adult. The negative is so often stressed in what I call the 'you know that chocolate isn't good for you syndrome.' We have been conditioned to expect less joy and fulfillment as we age, and so often we get what we expect! There are so many negative expectations of advancing in years! Culture has taught us to expect less as we age. It has taught us to see the limitations as definitive of who we are and what we can do and become. The aging know the limitations that come with the progression of years, what they often don't know is how to deal with those limitations. The 'silliness' is not something we often talk about. Why can't someone in their eighties or nineties laugh at their limitations, why can't they eat chocolate? Why can't older adults live with a certain abandon and freedom? Are we afraid they might get fat? Are we afraid they might enjoy the experience of aging? We need to laugh at the self-imposed limitations so that we are free to deal with the unchangeable limitations.

Humor, in ministry with/for the older adult is a necessary ingredient! It is one tool that allows us to offer abundant life where none is expected. Laughter brings healing and wholeness, if only for the moment. This is true both for the aging person and for the one caring for him.

When my mother was in the nursing home she had a roommate who was ninety five years old and quite ill. Every time I would visit my mother she would tell me about how sick Ruby was. So it was no surprise when I visited her one morning to help her eat her breakfast that she told me, with great sadness, that Ruby had died during the night. As I was consoling her I noticed out of the corner of my eye that Ruby was sitting up in bed enjoying her breakfast. "Mom, do you think you had a dream about Ruby? She obviously is alive and well?" Without batting an eyelash my mother looked over at Ruby's bed, saw she was alive, and said, "I'll be darned, she was dead last night." I could have scolded her for such a nonsensical response! I could have been depressed that she was so out of touch with reality! I could have tried to help her see how wrong she was! I could have had any number of responses. My choice was to smile and say, "Mom, you've always been right! God must not have wanted Ruby just yet." I laughed as I said it. She laughed at the situation and went on eating her breakfast as if nothing out of the ordinary had just taken place. Humor, well placed, used to defuse a situation and to enable an affirmation of life's joy was the tool that helped. In that moment she heard, at whatever level she was capable of hearing that God was in charge of our lives. She experienced acceptance and love, rather than criticism or correction. She experienced joy in what might have been a disturbing moment in her confusion. Humor had helped a difficult moment make sense, and it affirmed her as a person of value. What better reason to employ humor is there?

Ministry with and for older adults need not be humorless! In fact it is most effective when humor is part of the picture. It may be even more important for the care giver to learn to see the humor, the "silliness" of aging than it is for the older adult. Too many adult children and care givers are so caught up in their sympathy for the aging and cannot enjoy the moment they are in. This often leads to a weariness of caring, a 'burned out' feeling.

When a youngster says something foolish, we don't cry or get upset, we enjoy the moment. In fact there were moments when my children were younger that I wished the moment would freeze. The "silly" things they said and did had me laughing and brought me joy. As a grandparent I am recovering some of these moments as the grandchildren do and say "silly" things. I enjoy the moment and also recall so many such moments of the past and have a double enjoyment. We would do well to rediscover that sense of laughing in the present moments at the "silliness." Older people have enough seriousness in their lives already. "Laugh, love and live" still seems like a good maxim to follow.

How we use humor and when we use it hard to pin down. It can be used inappropriately! My rule of thumb is that humor is contextual. I must know the person before employing it. I must know what he or she finds funny or humorous. As I used to tell my children when they were young, something is not funny if the other person does not laugh. I do not use humor to make myself feel better. I only use it if it serves to relieve the other person's anxiety or stress and opens the door for seeing from a new perspective.

So do not be afraid of humor in such ministry, but always keep in mind the relational context. The person(s) receiving the humor must have a relationship with the one using it in order to receive it as loving and accepting. A case in point occurred at our Long Term Care building. Just as I was arriving for some visiting, one of the patients, having a behavioral issue common to many dementia patients, called a nurse to his side and attempted to feel her breasts. He wondered aloud "are they real?" Unacceptable behavior by any measure! The nurse had to make an immediate decision on how to stop the behavior. She could have justifiably scolded him, embarrassing and demeaning him! She could have simply moved away and walked on, leaving him alone and leaving, not addressing the issue. Instead she employed humor. She moved his hand, backed up, and said, "Look at me, would anyone pay to have them look like this?" He laughed, she laughed, and the situation was defused. His bad behavior was stopped without feeling put down. She was able to then say to him that his actions were not acceptable and that he could not behave that way again. Humor rightly used helped create a situation in which growth could happen, in which ministry could take place. That nurse could not have responded as she did if she did not already know the patient and have already been known by him as someone he could trust.

A story that speaks to using humor to defuse a tough situation that has personal significance for me occurred several years before going to the United Methodist Homes. As many adult children do, we had to place my mother into a Long Term Care facility when a stroke left her unable to stay with my family. For the most part she was accepting of that fact. Her social skills, despite a decline in cognition, stayed with her. She loved being with other residents most of the day. One day, however, her nurse said there was a problem. "We haven't mentioned it before because we thought it would resolve itself. Several days have passed and she refuses to leave her room. She says that every time she does the ducks nip her ankles. Now mind you, she was on the third floor of the building. There were no ducks there or anywhere in the building. There was no convincing her that there weren't any ducks. Even a conference with the staff could find no solution. A few days later my brother Tom came to see her. I shared the story with him. He laughed and said "I'll take care of it." And did! He went into her room, asked about the bothersome ducks, and repeated his statement. "I'll take care of it," and left the room. A few minutes later we began to hear a commotion outside her door. Bang! Pop! Gotcha! Residents were laughing at this crazy man with an imaginary rifle shooting at imaginary ducks. Nurses and aides were laughing. A good time was being had by all. Soon he came back to the room and announced, "You can leave your room again. I shot every duck. There are none left to bother you." My mother laughed and thanked him. The three of us went downstairs, sat outside and enjoyed a pleasant afternoon

Humor is a useful tool, but needs to be used carefully. It can never be effective if it is used as a weapon, is sarcastic, or misunderstood by the one hearing it! It has to be contextual. Just as a good comedian changes his material depending on the audience, so must we. The nature of the relationship and the situation determines the use of humor. Laughter is indeed good medicine! Older adults receive physical and psychological benefits from a good laugh as well as anyone else. It is seeing a partial person, rather than a whole one, that keeps much of our ministry so somber. A ministry of healing is one in which smiles and laughs should be as commonplace as one with tears and worry. Allowing people to rejoice in the "silliness" of aging is a gift not offered nearly enough. So explore ways in which good, healthy humor can be shared with the aging.

For Further Thought

Humor is a 'funny' thing! It can be used to enable a better vision of person's sense of self or of situations. It can be used in exactly the opposite way, denigrating a person and making a tough situation even worse.

Can you identify times when humor has helped you gain a new, more positive perspective? How did that happen for you?

Can you identify times when humor has hurt you? How did that happen for you?

Have you experienced older adults being hurt by someone else's idea of humor? Is it ever appropriate to use such humor?

This section contains a number of stories in which the author felt humor was appropriately used. What role did his relationship with the people involved play in making the humor appropriate? Can you imagine situations in which such humor would be inappropriate?

The author has a list of guidelines for using humor. Would you add anything to the list?

SEXUALITY AND
THE OLDER ADULT

One of the places where a good sense of humor is important is in this area of sexuality. An older adult does not cease having feelings, thoughts, and memories that are sexual in content. Being uptight and squeamish about this is not helpful, nor is being in denial. Seeing a whole person allows us to more readily recognize this fact as we do our ministry.

Many an older person acts out this reality in inappropriate ways, while some do so quite appropriately. Others either don't exhibit any concern in this area or simply sublimate that concern. I became increasingly aware of this at Wesley Village. Several of our residents were acting out as the man in the previous story did. There is a lot of hand holding, hugging, and flirting among the residents. I must admit I was initially surprised at this behavior. My bias about the aging was that such things were a part of their past, not their present. Rationally I knew better than that. I had been a pastor for forty years when I took this position. I had seen the same behavior before. I performed weddings for people in their eighties. Some of my older members dated frequently. Some lived together. There was no question that I knew better. But these folks, it seemed to me, were the exceptions. They were different than the rest. That is why they stood out.

The surprise was how often I witnessed behavior with a sexual content, how often I heard our residents share racy jokes, how often I heard them talking about other residents who were acting out their sexuality. We are not comfortable talking with our children about this subject and we certainly are not comfortable talking with the aging about this subject. As those engaged in a ministry of caring for the whole person, we do well to remember that sexuality is a part of creation. We know that it is life giving and we must discover ways to affirm it as such even among older adults. I do not pretend to have the answer to how we do so, but I do know it requires acknowledging the fact that the older adult, like every other human being, is sexual. Sexuality is a component of his/her wholeness. How she/he expresses it is as different as the individual and the situation. But that it will be expressed is without doubt! We do a real service to the aging when we find ways to discuss this subject from the vision of our faith. In large measure, we have not done that! One incident stands out as an example of inappropriate behavior which might have been a different event had conversations on sexuality and older adults been an openly accepted possibility. It led to the following article and thoughts.

"I need to talk with the two of you about what I saw today." And so began a very awkward, painful conversation! The participants were a man and a woman, both of whom were in the eighties and me. Because of my position I know all of our residents as well as anyone else on staff. So it seemed obvious that of all the people on our staff I was the likely one to initiate this conversation. What I had seen had been seen repeatedly by other staff and residents. All, including myself, were uncomfortable initiating this conversation. What had occurred on more than one occasion is that this 'couple' was engaged in our public areas in some very inappropriate sexual behavior (inappropriate, at least, in public).

When the conversation began, it was embarrassing to the couple and to me. Yet the situation had to be addressed. How it was addressed is less important than the reminder the situation presented. It is one we are often uncomfortable with and which we often deny. It is the reminder that older adults have the same urges and need to express their sexuality as younger people do. How that need is met is as different as the situation and as different as the individual involved. Coupled with this reminder, came the awareness that we are often in denial about this fact. We don't want to acknowledge that Mom or Dad or Grandma or Grandpa even think about such things.

Surely part of our sexuality seeks ways for physical touch. Studies continue to show that babies thrive best when they are touched and held. It is safe to say that is true for all people at every age of life. Finding ways for older people to satisfy this need is often problematic. That concern must have been in my mind when I found myself humming,

"You must remember this, a kiss is still a kiss, a sigh is still a sigh. The fundamental things apply as time goes by" These are words from the movie **Cassablanca.** They also apply to the aging population.

It is easy to forget that aging does not end a person's need for feeling loved, for feeling special, to sense that someone finds him or her warranting a 'kiss.' A kiss, a physical statement that says 'I love you' is never only a kiss or a physical statement. A kiss, a touch gives credence to any words of love we might say. As we age the intense passion of our younger years may diminish, but the need to be touched, the need to be specifically noticed by and special to someone does not. This is increasingly true "as time goes by," as our activities become more limited and our circle of family and friends grows smaller.

It is too easy for caregivers, pastors, lay visitors, and family members and friends to pay so much attention to the physical needs of those for whom they care to forget to pay attention to their emotional needs. It is too easy to forget that a necessary ingredient of a healing ministry is recognizing that saying we love someone is different than demonstrating that fact. Especially is it difficult to do so in socially appropriate ways.

I'm not sure how to deal with this in the context of my ministry with older adults, but I am sure that if I am not aware of it, I am not likely to address the needs of the whole person.

So, some preliminary thoughts!

1. Be willing to let the subject of sexuality in older adults be permissible. It is not a dirty subject. It is a human subject. It is part of creation.

2. Be aware that expressing one's sexuality at any age is about much more than 'sex.' It is about declaring 'I am human and I matter to someone.'

3. Take every opportunity to express the human need to be touched that seems comfortable to you and him/her. Hold a hand, give a hug, pat the shoulder, or put your arm on the person. (Only do any of these if the relationship is such that such action is acceptable and not going to be misunderstood.)

4. In an institutional setting (church, nursing home, assisted living facility) provide opportunities for people to express their need for physical contact in a socially acceptable, appropriate way. Rituals such as the passing of the peace and holding hands in a circle of prayer are both theologically correct and helpful ways to touch another human being. Dancing, for those able, is another possibility.)

Shortly after a resident dance, *The Senior Prom*, at one of our communities the importance of suggestion four was highlighted for me. Our activity director and several volunteers danced with the residents who wanted to do so, who had no other partner. Before the dance was over I noticed Louise watching the dancing from her wheelchair. It seemed to me that she had a wistful look on her face. I asked her to dance and she said she could not stand up. "I know that, but I bet you can dance anyway if you would allow me to lead you." I took hold of her hands, knowing she was strapped into the chair and would not fall out, and gently wheeled her around to the beat of the music. A simple thing to do, but as the commercial goes, it was priceless. Immediately after the dance, and for several days after, Louise told me and all her friends that that simple act had made her "feel like a woman" for the first time since she was confined to a wheelchair. In other words, she felt her sexuality had been affirmed.

Part of our wholeness is clearly found in finding ways to express our sexuality. A vibrant ministry with and for older adults will seek ways to allow this to happen.

For Further Thought

Discussing sexuality is often difficult. Many a parent has fretted over when and how to discuss the topic with his/her child. It is no less difficult to do so with an older adult. Especially is this so when we do not see people in that population as being concerned with such an issue. How comfortable are you with this topic in general, in terms of your parent(s), or any older adult?

If the situation warranted such a conversation in your ministry would you be willing to do so? If an adult child of an older adult approached you regarding a parent's acting out feelings of sexuality, how would you respond?

MEANINGFUL VISITS WITH OLDER ADULTS

All meaningful ministries take place within the context of relationships of trust. These relationships are built and nurtured over a period of time. Visiting one on one, getting to know each other is vital. But for many, doing so is a worrisome chore. What will we talk about? How will I get to the concern I have without being manipulative and without provoking frustration or anger? Suppose she does not want to talk? Real questions asked in countless ways by those engaged in caring for/about an older adult. Especially are they real for someone who has no prior experience with visiting older adults.

"I'm going to see Sally Brown and I don't know what to say. After all she is 95 years old and is showing signs of Alzheimer's disease. I'm only 33 and not used to being around people that old."

A common concern and a common fear! Is there a right way and a wrong way to visit a person such as Sally Brown? I don't think there is as long as the visitor is open and present to that person at that moment. People at any age have the need to be relational, to have a sense of value in someone else's eyes. Visit! Say hello! Express your gladness at the chance to be with that person! Notice the environment - the way the person is dressed, the photographs in the room, the knickknacks, etc. Enter that person's world by asking inviting questions. (Examples:

This is a beautiful photo, whose is it? I have a doll very similar to yours, how long have you had it? I always wondered about its history.) Let the one being visited set the agenda and the tone!

Asking to enter the other person's world is a sure way to signal the desire to know the person. It tells that person you are interested in her, that you want to take the time to listen. Well framed questions suggest a willingness to let the other person lead the conversation. He will sense that willingness and more likely allow you to enter his world to the extent he feels comfortable doing so. Open ended questions allow the one being visited to reply in ways that he finds appropriate. Much of the worry about conversing with older adults is based on a hidden assumption that they are less capable of doing so than younger people. I have not found that to be true at all! What I have found is that the aging often need more time to frame their thoughts than they once did and because of the sense that "no one has the time to wait for me to talk" they become less conversational. Like everyone else they have a need to talk about their lives - present and past! Like everyone else they have fears and dreams! Like everyone else they deal with all of these things much better if they can do so with a caring person! Visiting is an ideal way to establish relationships that will allow a person to reveal her deepest concerns, fears and joys. It begins the process of seeing beyond any limitation, mental or physical. It enables witnessing to a holistic gospel because it recognizes a whole person. In every one of my years in ordained ministry the most rewarding experiences have come out of trusting relationships born in a ministry of visitation, which is ultimately a ministry of listening. Visiting by pastors, lay people and family members can be cause for anxiety. They can also be cause for celebration and affirmation of the one being visited. What better result could there be from such efforts? What makes the difference?

Hear the story about Fred with this question in mind! It speaks to a common anxiety which feeds on itself and grows in intensity. It is the anxiety of wondering if we will know what to say at any given moment. And it is an anxiety that keeps many of us from effective visits not only with older adults, but with others as well.

Fred was an interesting guy. He was totally committed to his church. He was friendly and seemed to make conversation very easily. It was difficult to know him and not like him. He was talented in so many areas and appeared comfortable within himself. So it was a great surprise when I discovered that every time he and his wife invited people to their home for dinner (which they did very often) Fred would go into panic mode. Afraid he would not be able to carry the conversation, he would research the people coming. He would find their interests, carefully read the local newspaper and literally take notes on possible things to say and ways to keep the conversation going. I will never understand why this bright, caring, interesting guy felt so insecure. But he did and it made him ill-at-ease in such settings. When in other settings, he was perfectly comfortable and a joy to be with.

"Jim, I'd make that visit for the church, but I don't know what to say. I am not good around old people. Can you give me ideas about what to say?"

If I had a nickel for every such conversation (my Fred conversations) I'd be rich. It speaks to a basic insecurity about dealing with the unknown. My response has always been the same. "Would you plan a conversation with your Mom or grandmother? Go and be yourself. That is who they want to see and meet."

Visiting with older adults need not be a worrisome thing. It is a joy and actually quite easy. Older adults are no different than anyone else at any age.

They may be hard of hearing - but they still have a need to be heard.

They may have trouble seeing - but they still need to be seen.

They may be slow speaking - but they still need to speak.

What a gift we bring when we allow a visit to be free flowing, listening to the older adult and letting the conversation go where that person needs it to go.

What a joy we enable when we allow the older adult to be seen and heard, rather than a chore to be accomplished.

So if there is a Fred within you, banish him. Visit unencumbered by an agenda. Let the needs, the concerns, the joys, the sorrows of the moment lead the conversation. You will be enriched by knowing you truly visited with another person of worth and they will be also.

What made Fred so anxious? What makes others so anxious? I believe it is an underlying assumption that "If I don't carry the conversation, it may fall flat on its face." It is about controlling where and how the conversation will proceed. There is nothing sinister about this. It is not necessarily born of a desire to control, but rather of a fear of failing to engage in a meaningful conversation. It leads to a lack of listening, to a lack of picking up clues from the other person as to where the conversation might go. The anxiety can be eliminated if we begin the task of visiting with a different assumption. My assumption is that every person - regardless of age - has a story to tell. Which is to say: every person has plenty to say. I do not have to carry a conversation in order for it to succeed. I have to be open and ready to listen to what the other person has to say and tell. I have to assume that within the physical person in front of me is a whole person, able to share his thoughts and feelings as well as I am able to share mine. I might ask open ended questions, as noted earlier, but I have to enter a conversation willing to let it go where the other person wants it to go. Obviously there are times when visits are arranged to discuss specific issues. Even then, being open to hearing the other person makes the conversation flow more smoothly. When a person knows she is being heard, she is more able to hear the other person.

The assumptions we make determines the success or failure of our ministry of visitation. They determine the extent of our ability and desire to listen. Meaningful visits are times of intentional listening, something which too many older adults do not experience. Keeping the goal of seeing a whole person before us makes all the difference in this experience. Seeing the whole person creates an interest in learning who this person is, rather than what problems she has. Rather than beginning with the all too natural assumption that older people are limited and "need our help" meaningful visits and conversations begin with the assumption that older people have something important to contribute. We can banish the anxiety with this awareness and be constantly surprised when those we visit add to our understanding of life. Older adults have learned much along the way and are a resource for those who would seek to be in ministry with/to them. We tap this resource each time we engage in a listening ministry, the key element of which is visiting without an agenda. It takes time and effort for this type of ministry, but the rewards are significant!

For Further Thought

Visiting an older adult often causes anxiousness for the one visiting. Like Fred, the question of what to say is a concern. Suppose the person doesn't want to talk? Suppose I can't engage the person? Suppose I say the wrong thing? How comfortable are you in visiting an older person? Is there some of Fred in you?

The writer suggests that our assumption that we are responsible for the conversation and its contents is detrimental to a conversation. He suggests that a good conversation begins with a willingness to listen, enabled by asking to 'enter the other person's world." How do you understand what he is saying?

Have you ever had a person demonstrate the willingness to enter your world by asking about something important to you? Did that lead to a conversation that was more satisfying than others you have had?

What are some elements of a meaningful visit? Do you feel able to make such a visit?

Why? Why not?

SOME CONCLUDING THOUGHTS

She is ninety eight years old, is as sharp as tack, and recently joined one of our Assisted Living Communities. She charmed her way into my heart immediately. She is warm and radiates joy. "It is the best decision I have ever made" was her response to my question: "Are you adjusting to your new setting." "I'm just fine. People are wonderful here. They all care so much." "That is good to hear. Do you have any questions that I might be able to answer?" "Just one" was the answer. With a twinkle in her eye she asked:"Can you tell me why I've lived so long?" It was a question she answered for herself. "I guess you cannot. No one can! But so long as I am, I may as well make the most of it and enjoy it as best I can."

Oh that everyone had that attitude as they age! Oh that I keep that attitude! Ann raises the question, even as she answers it. What is the meaning and purpose of a ministry of caring for older adults? What is the essential task? Is it not, as she (without saying the words) has discovered about her later years. Is it not to create environments in which the aging person might discover the promise of new life? Is it not to provide a witness to abundant living, which is a promise without an expiration date? Is it not to challenge those for whom we care to see promise in each new day, to help them declare with Ann: "But as long as I'm alive, I may as well make the most of it and enjoy it as best I can?

We have to stop fearing challenging people as they age with the call and promise of the good news of abundant living and its availability to all. We must not be trite or blasé about the realities of aging, many of which are most unwelcome and not conducive to abundant living. We cannot let the aging off the hook, as it were, failing to remind them that even in the face of adversity, they are called to abundant living. Too often out of a misguided sense of compassion, we offer platitudes, rather than challenges to make the best of life and enjoy it. We often run the risk of downsizing the possibilities of growth and joy with statements, that in and of themselves are true, but appear hollow in tough moments of life. "Things will get better." The truth is they often will not and older adults know that! We promise a 'new life in the world to come,' when the need is for a way to live in the here and now. It is a disservice to our loved ones and those for whom we care not to challenge them to see the possibilities.

The point is this! Ministry with and for older adults is not always easy. The physical and cognitive failures which often accompany this age group make it difficult to see beyond. This lack of seeing beyond precludes being effective in offering a gospel of abundant life to a person called, even at advanced age, to wholeness. It lends itself to sympathy, rather than empathy, and allows us to forget the gospel's challenge to *"Come, follow me!"*

Recently I had lunch with colleagues who do ministry in one of our facilities. We were talking about how and what to preach in a nursing home. The comments speak volumes about the difficulty of being in ministry with and for older adults. And although we were discussing preaching in a nursing home, we all knew our focus was larger than that. For whether in a nursing home, a hospital, at home alone, or with a family member, the aging present a challenge for preachers, and by extension, for anyone seeking to care for him or her in a creative way.

One colleague said he always preached on one of two topics, forgiveness and hope. It was his contention that these were topics to which the people could relate since they were in a 'contrived setting' with roommates they would most likely not have chosen had there been a choice, being cared for by people they also would likely not have chosen to be their caregivers. He said such factors led to anger, often directed toward the roommates and caregivers, often misplaced anger at the fact of the need to be in such a situation in the first place. Forgiveness, he said, is relevant. "They need to forgive themselves and the others. They cannot hear this message often enough!" "Hope," he said, "is what they need as much as forgiveness. They need to know that something better is coming when this life is over."

Another said he always kept his sermons and liturgy 'light-hearted' since this age group usually experiences so much sadness and sickness. "They need to be lifted up, allowed to laugh and forget their situation for a while." Then he said, "I try not to challenge them, they have enough to face already!"

Still another said something that was music to my ears. "I try to offer the same message to the folks in Long Term Care as I do in my church. There is only one gospel! There is not a different message for one age group and another for others. I am cognizant of the situation, always aware of limitations, but I do not water down the gospel. These folks need to know, as much as you and I do, that God loves them, empowers them, and expects them to accept the gift of life no matter how it is wrapped. They need to be challenged to do all they can to love, care, and serve others.

My response was "Amen."

If we are to be in ministry with and for older adults we must see them in their wholeness and offer them a gospel message that will call them and inspire them to claim that wholeness even in the face of limitations, maybe even because of the limitations. We must move beyond the assumption that they are different than we are in terms of their spiritual needs. We must move beyond seeing anger, grief, loss and a host of other self-limiting experiences as the defining factor in a person's life. We must move beyond simply offering hope for the future, as important as that is, and also offer hope for the present, which is born of knowing the presence of God and the claim of God in the present moment. And we must move beyond using worship as entertainment, trivializing the content of a life-saving, life-giving gospel. Surely the worship experience for any age group can be enjoyable, even provide some good laughs, but if it is devoid of the challenge to become new persons, living as fully as possible in the present, rejoicing and relying on a loving, present God to do so, it is not worship!

While these are thoughts about preaching they also point the way to effective ministry for and with older adults on every level. This *'way'* is not about one way! There are many ways to be in ministry, many ways to share the gospel, This *'way'* is about seeing a person, seeing a soul, and responding to the need of that person, that soul. A voice from my past continues to speak to me about the basics of caring for and about older adults. It is Al's voice, a friend who died over forty years ago.

Less than two weeks out of seminary, at my first full time appointment as a pastor, Al came to see me. Al was fifty years my senior, a retired United Methodist minister, and more than ready to offer advice. Never was the advice offered meanly or critically. It always came with a sense of caring and was always welcomed. Over the years, we became good friends and colleagues with a great deal of respect for each other. In fact, Al visited me each Tuesday morning, even after I had moved sixty or seventy miles away from where he lived. He became part of the family, performing baptisms for our children, attending birthday parties and picnics. He saw our children as 'the children I never had.'

I've long wondered what it was that drew me to a true friendship with a man fifty years older than I. One thing is certain! The friendship began the very first day he visited me and offered advice. What prompted that advice that made me want to know him better?

Al clearly sensed that, as a young twenty-four year old newly graduated from seminary, and appointed to a congregation with a lot of older people, I was feeling a bit uneasy. In seminary there were no classes on how to win the trust of a much older generation. He said, "Jim, if we know you love us, you can do and say anything you want to. You can make all sorts of mistakes, and you will. (He was right on the money with that observation!) You don't even have to be a good preacher. The more you love us, the more your preaching will improve. In the final analysis, just love us. That's all anyone really wants or needs."

These words rang true instantly! I've carried them with me throughout my ministry. They have never been proven wrong. In fact when I practice them, they are always proven absolutely right. In those moments of ministry and caring, when doubtful of my ability to do or say the right thing, these words led the way. When I remembered 'just love' them the doubt disappeared and ministry happened. Against this backdrop the following guidelines are an attempt to capture this 'way' of doing ministry for and with the older adult, regardless the way you choose.

GUIDELINE FOR MINISTRY WITH OLDER ADULTS

One of the joys of my present position comes in the form of requests to share ways of enabling congregations to engage in such ministry. These come as requests for preaching, for speaking, and for conducting workshops. Having done so for several years I have come to expect a common question. It is the "how to" question. It is the question I am asked most frequently. It is not asked because congregations are not already doing such ministry. It is asked because they realize that so much more can be done with older adults than we are doing.

How do we begin a ministry with older adults? That is the question! My answer is fluid, for no one way is the only way. Every situation demands its unique response. This is true even if the question is asked by an individual or by a family member seeking to respond to the aging one they know and love. Rather than answer concretely, thereby suggesting a closed answer, I offer these guidelines. These guidelines summarize the previous discussions and articles. They are based in the theology that sees every human being as a valuable, unique, contributor to the global family. They are based in the theology that sees life as a gift to be lived as fully as possible regardless the circumstances of the moment. They assume that living life to the fullest is not possible if life becomes self-centered rather than relational and service oriented. And they are based on the conviction that too often we have overlooked the truth of these statements because we have accepted the premise that aging is a disease to be avoided until there is no other choice. They assume that much of our cultural conditioning and a misunderstanding of what it means to 'help someone' is incorrect and needs revisiting. My firm conviction is that helping someone may mean doing for them what they cannot do for self, but that most importantly it means fostering an atmosphere where they can reclaim autonomy and choice in their individual life and situation.

These guidelines are:

1. Be sure to ask the persons most affected by the ministry what they think! Anything less devalues them. It misses from the outset the goal of ministry to whole persons who have something to offer.

2. As much as possible, emphasize doing ministry 'with' rather than 'for' them. Allow them the opportunity to see themselves as important and capable.

3. Remember that all Christians have a call and a need to be of service to others. Older adults are no different than the rest of us in this regard. Explore ways in which they might still be of service to someone else regardless of frailty or illness.

4. Allow whatever ministry you create to uncover and enhance the specific gifts of the older adults included in this ministry.

5. Be creative! If your congregation (or you individually) have never done it that way before, that may be the reason to try it that way now.

6. Remember, it is not about having a program for older adults; it is about meeting the spiritual needs of older adults. These needs are human needs! They include:

   6.a The need to feel valued as a whole person, worthy of respect.

   6.b The need to be heard.

   6.c The need to be loved unconditionally

6.d The need to be involved in making choices about care, living arrangements and such.

These guidelines will produce an effective ministry with the older adults.

If I were to attempt to summarize my thoughts on ministry with and for older adults, it would be to say that the goal is to enable the individual to discover the gold in the "golden years. It is this belief that prompted the following sermon and many others like it that I give in response to the request to 'Come to my church and share a sermon on Ministry with the Older Adult.

Who Said They Were Golden Years?

II Corinthians 4:16 - 5:10

I got a call from my neighbor one day to tell me that she had company. I thought it was strange that she would call just to tell me that. But then she said, "Guess who it is?" I was stymied until my mother got on the phone and invited me to join them. She lived with me and had gone out for a walk, which she often did. On the way home she became confused, walked into the neighbor's house, which was laid out like mine, thought she was home and was making herself comfortable when my neighbor heard her. When I went to get her, she was indignant. She did not wish to go next door to my house, she wanted to stay in her own home and entertain.

We began to explore other options for my mother, as we became more aware of her advancing dementia. But as we struggled with what to do, my mother said to me, "Whoever said they were golden years? Then she added, "They are a lot more tarnished that I would have thought."

And so they were! And so they are! And so they will be!

I see that every day at Wesley Village, our United Methodist Homes facility in Shelton. As most of you know I am the Director of Spiritual Life there and, as such, I know the residents and many of their family members really well. What strikes me is how differently people deal with aging. Some seem to do it so graciously! Others make you want to cry when you see their frailty and infirmity! Others make you crazy with the griping and complaining, with nothing and no one satisfying them. Others make your day by the appreciation for anything that is done for them.

And I wonder, what makes the difference?

Reportedly, when John Quincy Adams was well beyond his expected life span a young friend met him on the street and asked, "How is John Quincy Adams today?" Adams reportedly answered, "John Quincy Adams is very well, thank you. But the house he lives in is sadly dilapidated. It is tottering on its foundations. The walls are badly shattered and the roof is worn. The building trembles with every wind and I think John Quincy Adams will have to move out before long. But he himself is very well, thank you."

Emerson said, "The years teach much which the days never know."

My mother, even as her condition progressed, would always say of her situation, "It could be worse. I still have my life." I would think to myself, tarnish and all.

Were they onto something?

I think they were!

Making peace with aging, making peace with one's own mortality sets a person free to be who she is, who he is! Some days I cannot help thinking that the folk with whom I work and minister would uniformly fare better if they and their families would face the realities before them. How often I want to remind them of the gospel message that "the truth will set you free."

The truth is that all of us begin to age the moment we are born. The truth is that the overwhelming number of us will live longer than our parents did, and that most of us will find our bodies and our minds diminishing in ability as we advance in years.

So how do we do that gracefully? How do we do that faithfully? How do we reach the point my friend Lurie reached recently?

She was currently a patient at Wicke Health Center and asked her family to call me and ask me to come visit her that day. I got there and her daughter met me in the hallway, obviously upset and teary.

"My mom has decided to die and wants to talk to you."

Now I knew Lurie had serious health issues and that she was ninety one years old, so the news was not totally unexpected. Nor was the conversation we had that morning. I knew her attitude about such things, having discussed them with her several times.

"Jim, I've asked to go on hospice care. I know I'm not getting any better. I know this disease is going to win. I don't want to pretend the medicine is helping, when it isn't. I'm ready to die. I've had a good life. I have no complaints. God has been good to me."

We talked for a while, held hands and said a prayer, seeking God's strength for her and her family as they faced the truth. A little over a day later, Lurie died peacefully.

What I have not told you about her is that she was wed to another resident the day after Christmas, both of them knowing how sick she was. Some friends and family thought it was so sad that she would die so soon after. She did not! She told me as she talked about her then up-coming wedding, "Life is for living, not for waiting to die."

How do we reach that state of faith, that state of grace - willing to live life to its fullest, all the while accepting death?

Adams, Emerson, thoughts of my mother, Lurie, all sent me back to our reading from II Corinthians this morning. Against the backdrop of these stories I ask you to listen to it, seeking in it a word from God, seeking in it a word of direction, finding in it a word of hope, a word of life.

"So we do not lose heart. Even though our outer nature is wasting away, our inner nature is being renewed day by day. For this slight momentary affliction is preparing us for an eternal weight of glory beyond all measure, because we look not at what can be see but at what cannot be seen; for what can be seen is temporary, but what cannot be seen is eternal.

"For we know that if the earthly tent we live is destroyed, we have a building from God, a house not made with hands, eternal in the heavens.... So we are always confident; even though we know that while we are at home in the body we are away from the Lord - for we walk by faith, not by sight. Yes, we do have confidence, and we would rather be away from the body and at home with the Lord. So whether we are at home or away, we make it our aim to please him."

How do we live with such grace?

How do we live with such faith?

How do we embrace life even as our bodies and our minds begin to fail us?

"We walk by faith, not by sight."

We affirm that the God who is responsible for us is Spirit and that if we are made in the divine image then, at the last, we too are Spirit. How often I have seen the truth of this insight! How often I have stood at the bedside of someone who has been ravaged by physical and mental ailments and heard a relative say, "You didn't know Mom when she was young, but even now there is an unmistakable presence about her that is the real Mom."

I suppose what they were trying to say is what I was trying to teach my confirmation classes about being spirit. I would ask them who I was. They would say, "Mr. Stinson"

or "Jim" or some nickname they had given me. I would then ask them: Who I would be if I had an arm amputated? They would answer,: "Mr. Stinson with one arm." "How about if I had both arms and both legs amputated?" With growing frustration they would note that I would still be Mr. Stinson. "What if my eyes were gone?" And so the game would go! Fairly soon one of the kids would inevitably say, "Mr. Stinson has a body, he isn't a body. There is something about him we cannot amputate."

As clumsy as that analogy is, it gives us the picture. We are more than a body; we are more than our physical selves. Any couple married long enough for age to set in knows that. Long after the initial physical attraction is but a memory, the attraction is still there, for lovers come to know something other than the body, they come to know the spirit.

All of which is to answer my mother's rhetorical question. "Who said they were golden years?"

God did!

God chose for us to have a body, even as Jesus had body. But more, God chose for us to be more than body, God chose for us to be spirit. And that has serious implications, especially in a culture that talks so much about body and so very little about spirit.

As people of God, as people who recognize we are spirit, we see the world differently than anyone else does. We deal with our lives differently than others. We relate to all others as spirit, as the presence of God. As such we don't war with others, for to do so is to war with God. We don't cast off others as if they do not matter, for to do so is to cast off God. We affirm our bonds by feeding the hungry, by housing the homeless, by relieving the oppressed, for not to do so is to leave God hungry and homeless, to leave God in bondage.

As people of God, as people who recognize we are spirit, we face the passing of time differently than others. We affirm it as part of the process that leads to a fuller awareness of the Spirit God, who gave us birth to begin with.

"Who said they were golden years?"

God did!

Ultimately life is golden, for life to the degree that it knows itself as spirit knows itself as the handiwork and presence of God.

They are golden when we are first held by a loving spirit, called parent.

They are golden in the teens when we are nurtured and loved by anxious and concerned spirits called Mom and Dad.

They are golden when we experience the downward spiral of our bodies, when they are touched and cared for by loving spirits called nurses, aides, and the like.

They are golden because they are God given, and God loved, and God inhabited.

"So we are always confident….." No matter what happens to our bodies "we are always confident."

Why? "It is because "we walk by faith, not by sight." Because we do we embrace all of life, even aging, even dying. For we know the body will die, but the spirit is forever!

WISDOM FROM AGING FRIENDS

Assorted Essays

Much of what I have learned about serving older adults has come about through the experiences I have been privileged to share with them. Book learning and classroom teaching can only go so far. Being present and willing to listen to their stories is what makes a ministry with this population meaningful and effective. The lives they have lived, and are living, are filled with wisdom and direction for those of us engaged in caring for and about them. Hearing their stories, their experiences, their joys and their sorrows, their successes and their failures is where effective ministry begins. It builds the relationships necessary to interact on any meaningful level with them No one book is sufficient to tell even the stories I have heard. Everyone has a story. Hence the infinite number of ways individuals age and deal with their lives.

The following essays are among the hundreds I have written over the years, most of which have not made it onto these pages. They are included because they did not seem to fit within the framework of this book, but nonetheless contain wisdom within them that is worth pondering. As all the essays in this book, they are based on real people with real experiences who, in telling their stories, have caused me to clarify my thoughts and behaviors. May they do the same for you!

- 1 -

Sarah died the other day. At 95 years of age, her last spoken words were:"I want to go home!" Her daughter learned over to her and said, "Mom, it's okay to go home. We'll be okay here. Go home! It was a poignant moment, followed very shortly by Sarah's last breath. It was especially poignant because she had lived at the Bishop Wicke Health Center for the last two years. During this time, every conversation with her began and ended with, "I want to go home. Why can't I go home?" No amount of comforting, no heroic efforts to help her feel at home worked for long. She might settle down for a while and enjoy her surroundings, seemingly participating in the events all around her. But the peace never lasted for long. Despite the fact that her family was very supportive of her, some members were there every day she still felt like a stranger. I often thought of the words, "Sometimes I feel like a motherless child a long way from home." I often try to relate to that sense of being lost and alone. It is a sense of many as they age. The ones who meant the most to them have often died, leaving a void. Their abilities, physical and mental often has decreased; their spirituality often has changed as questions begin to outweigh the traditional answers to which they have grown accustomed. It is a strange land. It does not feel like home. Sarah's plaintive cries to "Let me go home" are the cries of many people as they advance in age.

The challenge is to hear those cries as real, not just as ramblings of a confused old person." The challenge is to grow comfortable listening to the cries, allowing one self to feel empathy with the one expressing such feelings. The need to speak of these things aloud is very real, as is the need for someone to listen. As those who minister to/with older adults this is especially challenging. We so want to "fix" what is hurting someone. We want the pain to go away. In fact our work is not about "fixing" anyone, correcting what we see as imperfections, or as too negative. Our task is to listen empathetically, not always offering answers, but rather offering tenderness and caring. In my daily ministry, I've seen pastors, family members, and other caregivers negate the older person's real feelings. "You're just being foolish." "You don't really mean that." "I get upset when you talk that way."

We are called to be present to those with who whom we minister. We can witness to our faith and hope by truly listening. When someone knows they have been heard, spiritual healing begins to take place. People who feel accepted for who they are and what they feel often become less focused on their "own issues," becoming more engaged in what is going on around them. People who know they have been heard feel like they belong, feel like they are home. With Sarah, there are days when I just want to go home, figuratively and literally. That is not a negative thought in and of its self. It is a simple statement of need – need for a place and for people who allow me to say and be who I am – need for Home. Thank you Sarah for reminding there is a better way to be in ministry with older adults.

- 2 -

Rowena was by far one of my more memorable parishioners. She was always dressed in the latest style, always had her hair perfectly coiffed, was always open to new ideas, always able to deal with anything that life brought with it! I valued her input on various committees because she would always "cut to the chase," and insist that we deal with whatever issue was before us. She was never unkind, but spoke what she saw to be the truth, even if her friends disagreed with her. I loved conversing with her because her mind was so alive and active. Therefore I was surprised one day when this ninety plus year old woman showed me her driver's license, which had just been renewed. Where the awful photo that is usually there was supposed to be there was a beautiful photo of her when she was much younger. She had cut it out to fit over the Motor Vehicle picture, which she said made her "look like an old lady." "I don't see myself as an old lady and I don't expect anyone else to see me that way either." You had to love Rowena!

Perception is everything – or so it is said. Facts, for some of us, do not seem to get in the way of our preferred visions.

I thought of this recently when talking with one of the newer residents at Wesley Village. I had never met her before, but since this is a retirement village, I assumed that she was an older adult (which, by the way, she is). One of the first things she said in our first meeting was, "I am not now, and never will be, an older adult." She was vehement! I had never said anything about her age, but she clearly wanted me to know how she felt. In subsequent conversations the source of such feeling became clear. She had a preconceived notion of what our culture means when it uses such words (older adult, senior citizen, mature adult) and she did not and would not share the vision. More importantly, her family members had bought into the vision and were often trying to limit her in ways that she found inappropriate and based on a false vision of what getting older means. She and her family are not alone!

It is important that those of us who minister to and with older adults remember to check our assumptions!

The fact is that all people do not age the same way.

The fact is that – as with people of every age – variations are the rule not the exception.

The fact is that we, by virtue of living in a time and culture that idolizes youthfulness and seeks to prolong it as long as possible, have learned to see aging through a seriously warped vision.

The fact is that we need to examine our perceptions and allow each individual to be the unique event she is, the one of a kind creation he is, rather than seeing older adults as a monolithic package. Our ministry will become more creative, more individually focused, and more relevant as a result. We do ourselves and those we seek to minister to and with older adults as disservice if we do not.

She will be ninety-nine in July. If she told you she was seventy-five, you would have no reason to doubt her word. She is impeccably dressed at all times, her hair is perfectly coiffed and her nails are manicured and polished. She is striking in her appearance. What is most striking, however, is what accounts for her appearance. In one word, it is **attitude**. She has many of the frailties of a person her age. Dependent on a walker, occasionally forgetful and confused, she is, nonetheless, positively inquisitive, still questioning, still willing to try new things, reveling in her painting classes and engaging with everyone she meets. I look forward to visits with her because she exudes a zest for living.

In the past few years she has given up her condo, moved to assisted living and very recently been hospitalized and subsequently spent a couple of months at the Bishop Wicke Health Center in Shelton, CT. While she was there, her family, with her knowledge and permission, moved her to Wesley Heights, which is less expensive than Crosby Commons. Even though these moves were all on the same campus of the United Methodist Homes, they required upset and change to her routine.

Today, just before sitting down to write, her family brought her to see her new apartment for the first time. She'll be leaving the Health Center in a few days. Unlike a more common response to this type of change, true to the **attitude** we've come to expect from her, she said: **"I can't wait to see my new apartment. I'm so lucky! Who else, at my age, has the chance to start over?"**

The attitude is one of optimism, of hopefulness, of anticipation. Sound familiar? Aren't these at the very core of Christian faith? Aren't these a large part of what Jesus taught would be prevalent in the Kingdom of God? Should these not be part and parcel of our ministry to/with older adults? Should we not be challenging them and inviting them to engage their lives armed with these faithful traits? What better way to face the uncertainties, the upheavals and the frailties that often accompany us on our journey into aging?

Jesus does not promise the Kingdom of God and the peace that passes all understanding only to those below a certain age. He offers it to all who will accept its possibility and live accordingly – that is optimistically, hopefully and filled with anticipation of God's continuing presence in the twists and turns of our lives even to our dying moments. Our ministry to/with older adults, to be authentic, must be one of challenging them to faithfully live each day believing God still has something for them to do and to become. Anything less is not the Gospel! Anything less easily lapses into a ministry of pity and low expectations. Anything less dismisses the possibility of new life, of **the chance to start over.**

- 4 -

She is 98 years old, sharp as a tack, and recently came to Crosby Commons, our Assisted Living Community. She has been with us for less than two months so far. I had a delightful conversation with her and was charmed. There is a warmth and sense of joy radiating from her. "It's the best decision I ever made," was her answer to the question: "Are you getting adjusted?" "I'm just fine. People are wonderful here. They all care so much." "That is good to hear! Do you have any concerns or questions that I might answer?" "Just one," was the answer that was accompanied by a smile and a twinkle, "can you tell me why I've lived this long?" It was a question she answered for herself. "I guess you cannot. No one can. But so long as I'm alive, I may as well make the most of it and enjoy it as best as I can."

Oh that everyone had that attitude, especially as they age! Oh that I keep that attitude! That conversation with Millie got me thinking again about the meaning of being in ministry with older adults, and with the question we ask so often on the Conference Older Adult Ministry Committee. What is the essential task before us, before anyone, engaged in this particular ministry? Millie unwittingly answered it. Is it not to create environments in which people might discover the promise of new life (even in old age)? Is it not to provide witness to the Gospel's promise of abundant living (which doesn't seem to be issued with an expiration date)? Is it not to challenge the older adults with whom we are in ministry to see the promise of each new day, to call them to declare as she declares: "But so long as I'm alive, I may as well make the most of it and enjoy it as best I can"?

Too often we are fearful of challenging people as they age with the call and the promise of the Gospel, the call and the promise of abundant living. We are concerned with being seen as trite or blasé about the realities of aging, many of which are most unwelcome, and not conducive to abundant living. We let older people off the hook, as it were, on the call to live abundantly even in the face of adversity. Often out of a misguided sense of compassion. We denigrate the call to new life, with promises of "things will get better," or "in the hereafter, you'll be rewarded," which may be true, but which misses the present nature of the promise. "Come to me all who labor and I will give you rest." I have come that you may have life that is abundant." We do our elders a disservice when we do not challenge them to experience new life in the here and now, to see the God of life and abundant living in the midst of limitations.

There is no one way to create environments in which that call can be herd and received. We all have to wrestle with its implications. But hear Millie, feel the joy discovered in knowing that she doesn't have to have answers in order to live fully. Witness by your actions, your programming, your approach to the aging, that life can and should be lived as well (as fully) as possible. Witness to your faith, letting God lead the older adult to hear the call and the promise.

- 5 -

"Good morning!"

"What's good about it?"

And so began a conversation a few weeks ago with one of the residents of Wesley Village. Sitting at the table with three women she considers friends, eating a breakfast that might be served by a four or five star restaurant, having no significant health issues other than the all too predictable arthritis and various aches common in the older adult population, having family and friends visit her often, she still said, "What's good about it?"

Her reply did not stun me. She has often been a 'complainer.' Seemingly nothing is ever what she wants it to be. Her family has learned to live with her negative attitudes, saying, "She was not always this way. She got that way as she aged." They have accepted her negative attitudes and comments as part and parcel of the aging process. So it came as a surprise that when she asked me the question I responded with the unexpected. Knowing her and her tablemates well, and having used the same response with others, I took a chance and said in response to her question, "This is the day the Lord has made." The woman looked at me perplexed and then looked at her friends who replied in unison, "Let us rejoice and be glad in it."

She finally said to her friends, "What did you say?" With more emphasis this time, they repeated, "This is the day the Lord has made. Let us rejoice and be glad in it." I could not have been more pleased! It was almost as if I had planted their response. I did not! The result? She stopped by my office after breakfast and asked to talk. We did and she left saying "I don't mean to be so negative. I have so much going for me. It is just that I miss my old way of life. But I'm going to try to concentrate on what I have now, rather than what I do not have." Surely God must have smiled at that moment.

She is a constant reminder to all of us engaged in ministry with/ to older adults. The Church is called to witness to good news no matter where or what the circumstance. The Church has good news for everyone, including the older adults, who often forget the many gifts and blessings still available to them, not the least of which is the gift of life with all its limitations and frailties. Our task is to listen to the complaints as it were, and then to open the opportunity for the complainer to move beyond the negatives and begin seeing and enjoying the positives.

A reporter was interviewing a 104 year old woman: "And what do you think is the best thing about being 104?" She replied, "No peer pressure."

It was a humorous response? But much more than that! It reveals a deeper truth about aging. It is the inevitable loss of family and friends who helped define the person's sense of self and belonging in the world. One of the most common comments I hear from older adults can be summed up in a poignant comment my mother made several years before she died. "I know more people 'up there' than I do 'down here' these days." That is a truth people who reach old age know all too well. Loss is a common theme in their reminiscing.

Anyone doing ministry with older adults will most likely share the same observation. Some people seem to cope well with loss, moving on, regrouping, redefining the all-important sense of self and belonging, continuing to stay involved in life. Others seem to get stuck in their losses. Unresolved grief is a common phenomenon! We miss it too often, assuming 'old people' are just cranky, difficult to please, and other such negative assumptions. When we do so, we often miss a golden opportunity to minister in a life affirming way. I have heard many adult children scold their mother of father. "You "ought" to invite friends in!" "You "ought" to take part in more activities rather than sitting in your room all day." The list could go on. The "oughts" miss the point. My experience suggests that older adults already know they 'should' do these things, but just do not have the energy necessary to do so. That lack of energy often disappears when they are allowed to express the continuing pain of loss.

One of my greatest joys is seeing some resident emerge from the grief and move back into life. Often that happens after I, or someone else on our staff at United Methodist Homes, have sat patiently and listened to that resident's life story, including all the losses, releasing, in the telling of that story, the pain. How often a resident has said: "I haven't said anything like that in years. My family was tired of hearing me repeat the same story, so I just stopped telling it." Telling the story is a need of people in grief. When we don't recognize it in older adults, we are likely to get frustrated and more importantly, we are bound to miss an opportunity to enable new life to be found.

Listening! Enabling story telling! Growing comfortable with repetitions! These are all ingredients of a vital ministry with older adults.

- 7 -

Some years ago Elizabeth Kubler Ross wrote a book, <u>To Live Until We Say Goodbye</u>. It was a photo journal of people with terminal illnesses who allowed her to document the way they spent their last days. It was a beautiful book, giving the reader a glimpse into seeing death from a new perspective, and therefore seeing life from that same new perspective. The book vividly showed people living full, creative lives right up until the moment of their dying.

I thought of this book the other day when I received word that Esther had died. Esther was 95, a retired congregational minister, who lived at the United Methodist Homes in Shelton, CT. She was one of my favorite people. She read and discussed all the most recent books in theology, she pushed us as a community to be more ecologically involved, she struggled with contemporary issues trying to decide what response was the most Christian, studied the Bible with an open mind and spirit, constantly sought new insight, and truly loved and lived her life right up until the last moment.

I will, and already do, miss her greatly. She was a unique gift to the world. Indeed she was a unique gift to me. Her life was, and will remain, a constant reminder of a truth to remember as we do ministry with and for older adults. Simply put – Value their gifts! Allow those gifts to be used! More to the point perhaps is the flip side of these positive statements. Do not infantilize the older adult! She is always more than an illness or an infirmity! Do not assume the older adult cannot be challenged to grow! He is always able to see life as a gift to be used as fully as possible!

All older adults may not have the intellectual capacity or curiosity with which Esther was endowed, but they can grow – even in the most difficult circumstances. Allow your ministry with and for them to challenge them to accept the gospel call to abundant living even in their senior years. Simply keeping them busy is demeaning and unproductive. Struggle to create ministries of service and of new experiences. How you create such ministries will be as different as the person or group with whom you work! Not to do so is to miss an opportunity to put flesh on the call to abundant living!

Older adults are often sidelined by the inevitability of aging. The church needs to faithfully keep the vision of God in Jesus before us. God always sees beyond the limitations and sees a wholeness that we must accept for ourselves and which we must always offer to the older adult.

- 8 -

Two separate visits to two new residents at our assisted living facility at the United Methodist Homes on the same morning! They both arrived on the same day and now live a few doors from each other, never having met before. The contrast could not have been more extreme. Two distinctly different responses! Two radically different approaches to change!

One hopeful and expectant! One despairing and resigned to things never being any better! Both are suggestive of attitudes we bring to aging, whether our own or that of someone we care for and about!

Asked how things were going in their first week in a new setting, he said, "Couldn't be any better! I'm as free as a bird. I have my apartment and laundry cleaned for me, my meals are served and they're delicious. I can pick and choose from a variety of things to do! I go to my office at least once a week and do what I like the best – pursue my lifelong career." He is a mere 93 years old! She said, "I'm in prison! But what did I expect? Everyone gets old and this is what happens. I'll get used to it, but I'll never like it!" She is barely seventy years old!

Both attitudes, both approaches to aging are real in the older adult population. Both are real among those who do ministry with older adults. The first, obviously, is the more constructive and life giving. The second is self-destructive and saps the energy out of the person and those around him or her. The question these attitudes raise for those who care for and about older adults is, "Can I do something to foster the first and diminish the second?" Ultimately there is the frustrating reality that no one can change anyone else's attitude. Every individual is finally in charge of his or her attitude and approach to life. However there are some things that can help foster the possibility of a healthier attitude. Let me suggest a few. Listen, without judgment to the negative comments. Explore the reasons for the negativity. Often there are legitimate reasons for them. Talking about them and dealing with them often is therapeutic and helpful. After listening, gently observe some positive things, some concrete actions that might be taken.

   a. You used to love to knit, would you please make Mary a scarf? She would love one from you.
   b. Josie cannot see to read her own mail, you're a great reader, would you read to her?

Gently remind the person you care about of the strength and resilience he already has by having made it into being an older adult. That strength can still be tapped. Talk about spiritual resources that she might use. Expect a different attitude and share with her how much confidence you have that she will choose a different approach.

- 9 -

He had a major operation recently. Before surgery, his doctor told him that there was a good chance that he would end up with some paralysis. He said he prayed that any paralysis would not affect his arms and hands. In fact he did end up having full use of both his arms and hands, although he does have some paralysis of his legs. He did rehab as a patient at our Bishop Wicke Health Care Center. Every day he was there, he would leave his therapy sessions and play the piano in our lobby. The residents and visitors loved it and began asking what time he would be there each day. When it was time for him to go home he was asked if he had any questions. He had one! "May I come back as a volunteer and entertain when I am able?"

Great Spirit! Exemplifies an attitude of embracing all of life as a gift to be embraced! He told me: "God gave me this gift of music. I want to continue o share it for as long as I am able. God left me here. I believe my music is the reason."

To some, his theology may be problematic. But the spirit, the attitude is not! While we have breath, we have life, which is to say, we have a gift. It may be limited or different than it once was, but the gift of life was meant to be shared. For those of us engaged in ministry with and to older adults, delivering this message may be the most difficult of all. Aging often brings sickness, frailty and the life, which often results in a kind of paralysis. We hear hints of this paralysis every time someone says, in despairing tones, "I can't do what I used to do." Or, "Why does God leave me here?" The challenge before us for those engaged with older adults is offering a different vision. It is offering the vision of our faith, the vision of full and joyful life, the vision of purpose and meaning. I have seen the tremendous growth and joy of some of our most limited, challenged residents, even as I've seen some of our residents far less limited and challenged go from giving, caring people to self absorbed, unhappy people. In every instance the difference is having heard or not having heard the message. "God left me here. I believe my music is the reason."

Obviously the individual gifts vary! But I've yet to meet anyone who could not express (verbally or otherwise) the gift of love. I've yet to meet anyone who could not 'enjoy' some aspect of life and thus be a witness to the ongoing meaning of life. My observation (for whatever it is worth) is this. Many of us, out of a false sense of compassion, do not challenge despair among the aging as a lack of faith. We feel that to do so would be cruel. I have come to believe exactly the opposite! Not to offer the other vision is cruel, never calling the person to embrace the life that is, rather than the life that was.

So thank you my friend! I hope you are around when I get to the place where "I can't do what I used to do." I hope someone reminds me "God left me here." I hope someone calls me to say, "I believe my music is the reason."

I was having difficulty living alone, but did not want to live with my children. My wife had died, the house had become too big for me, and my kids live out of state. So I made the decision to come to United Methodist Homes, not saying "Gee how glad I am to leave my life behind, but saying what choice do I have?" These words speak to the observation attributed to Billy Graham who at age 87 said, "All my life I've been taught how to die, but no one ever taught me how to grow old." Philip was struggling with the question implied by Billy Graham. How do I grow old? Where do I go for help? Is there someone who can teach me how to deal with this phase of my life? Philip is another reminder that no matter how much we might want to deny it, the time of aging often brings unwanted changes, diminishing abilities, changes in mental status and a variety of other ailments. In a culture that urges financial preparation for the retirement years and pushes age denying panaceas, and all kinds of treatments and gimmicks to keep us feeling and looking younger than we are, there is often not adequate preparation for the realities of growing old. How many times I have heard adult children say, "If only mother has exercised more, if only Dad had eaten better and other such wishful thinking they might not have had to make these changes." Our culture has suggested in so many ways that we do not have to grow old. If we would just do the right things, aging would be a thing of the past. While practicing healthy living is desirable for people of any age, there is only one way to avoid growing old, exercise and good habits notwithstanding. It is called dying. Short of that as a goal, there is a need to help people grow old.

Our churches are in a strong position to do just that. It involves preaching and teaching the value of every living being. It involves telling the truth as made known by our Creator God. In doing so it means seeing all of life, in all its phases as part of the creative plan. The Church sees life on earth as linear rather than circular. Aging is one of the phases along this line. It is no less a phase than toddlerhood or adolescence. It is not something to be ignored by wishing "it will not happen to me or the ones I love." It is a phase that deserves understanding and acceptance. Just as a wise parent learns to cope with these other phases, allowing for the reality of the "terrible twos," or the reality of teen behaviors, adjusting to their limitations and needs, we need to help prepare our older adults, and all members of our congregations, to grow old with grace. The problem seems to be there are no rulebooks. There are, however, generalities that can be adapted for each individual situation and purpose.

Dignity!

Older adults want to be treated with dignity. They do not want to be treated like infants.

Independence!

Despite limitations, older adults want to retain as much independence as possible.

Choice!

Older adults, if cognitively able, need to make their own choices, even when adult children or other caregivers disagree.

Congregations have a role to play in teaching people how to grow old. Basic Christian values (unconditional love, including forgiveness and non-judgmental approaches to care) will help them find the way.

CPSIA information can be obtained at www.ICGtesting.com
Printed in the USA
BVOW09s0317270214

346174BV00001B/2/P